PRAISE FO

"Open monogamy is the #1 topic on so many of my patients' minds and is fast redefining what it means to be a couple. Whether you're curious, contemplating, or creating an open monogamy plan, I can think of no one better than Tammy Nelson to guide you every step of the way through the peaks and valleys of your journey."

IAN KERNER, PHD, LMFT

New York Times bestselling author of *She Comes First*

"Tammy Nelson has provided us with a hopeful, practical, and realistic guide to creating honest, values-led, flexible relationship agreements. With exercises, conversation guides, and stories from real life and the therapy room, she illuminates infinite possibilities for crafting unique and flexible forms of monogamy."

MARTHA KAUPPI, LMFT, CST-S

author of *Polyamory: A Clinical Toolkit for Therapists (and Their Clients)*

"Dr. Tammy Nelson's newest book, *Open Monogamy*, updates conceptions of monogamy to include the many different ways people relate today. With wit and compassion, and informed by decades of experience, Nelson guides readers through a deep consideration of how to build their ideal relationship. *Open Monogamy* provides thoughtful and useful guidance that is easy to understand and refreshingly free of judgment."

DR. ELISABETH SHEFF

author of *The Polyamorists Next Door, Stories from the Polycule, When Someone You Love Is Polyamorous,* and *Children in Polyamorous Families*

"When you agree to become monogamous, you agree to exile the parts of you that want something more or different than what your partner can offer. Many are willing to make this sacrifice in return for the sense of security that comes from restricting their partner's access to others. That restricting itself, however, can jeopardize relationships because those exiled parts don't disappear and, instead, may grow in influence over time.

"In this well-written and researched book, Tammy Nelson offers her years of experience helping couples navigate the turbulent waters of reappraising their commitments and potentially opening their relationships. Her sage advice is comprehensive, covering the pleasures as well as the pitfalls of taking such steps, and individualized—'opening' has many meanings and includes a spectrum of behaviors. If you are considering such a move, you won't find better guidance!"

RICHARD SCHWARTZ, PHD

developer of the Internal Family Systems model and author of *No Bad Parts*

"*Open Monogamy* provides a unique, creative road map for expanding your relationship in a healthy and honest way. Drawing on the experience of real couples, it provides expert advice and concrete exercises to help you live a life of passion while being true to yourself and those you love."

JANIS ABRAHMS SPRING, PHD

author of *After the Affair* and *How Can I Forgive You?*

"Dr. Tammy Nelson is not just a brilliant sex and relationship educator, sought-after international speaker, and extraordinary author but also a forward-thinking thought leader in today's sexual revolution. In *Open Monogamy*, she guides and supports you and your partner to make the rules on your terms so you can stay together in a committed and healthy way while exploring other options in the bedroom, instead of just fantasizing about it. She makes this delicate conversation shameless. I love learning from Dr. Tammy and so will you!"

DR. SHERRY ROSS

author of *She-ology* and *She-ology: The She-quel* and
cohost of the television series *Lady Parts*

"Dr. Tammy Nelson is a relationship revolutionary. Her rethinking of monogamy—as a practice, a continuum, and a flexible concept—is on point, actionable, and nothing less than a significant cultural shift. With *Open Monogamy*, she is back to blow minds and enhance partnerships."

WEDNESDAY MARTIN, PHD

New York Times bestselling author of *Primates of Park Avenue* and

Open
Monogamy

Open Monogamy

A GUIDE TO

CO-CREATING
YOUR IDEAL
RELATIONSHIP
AGREEMENT

Tammy Nelson, PhD

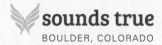
sounds true
BOULDER, COLORADO

Sounds True
Boulder, CO 80306

Published 2021

Cover design by Jennifer Miles
Book design by Linsey Dodaro

The wood used to produce this book is from
Forest Stewardship Council (FSC) certified forests,
recycled materials, or controlled wood.

Printed in the United States of America

BK06162

Library of Congress Cataloging-in-Publication Data
Names: Nelson, Tammy, author.
Title: Open monogamy : a guide to co-creating your ideal relationship
    agreement / by Tammy Nelson, PhD.
Description: Boulder, CO : Sounds True, 2021. | Includes bibliographical
    references.
Identifiers: LCCN 2021019958 (print) | LCCN 2021019959 (ebook) |
    ISBN 9781683647461 (trade paperback) | ISBN 9781683647478
    (ebook)
Subjects: LCSH: Non-monogamous relationships.
Classification: LCC HQ980 .N45 2021 (print) | LCC HQ980 (ebook)
    | DDC 306.84/23–dc23
LC record available at https://lccn.loc.gov/2021019958
LC ebook record available at https://lccn.loc.gov/2021019959

10 9 8 7 6 5 4 3 2 1

This book is dedicated to my husband Bruce and
to all our friends who make our lives exciting.

TABLE OF CONTENTS

NOTE TO READERS   xiii

INTRODUCTION **The Relationship of Your Dreams**   1

CHAPTER ONE   **Expanding Your Love**   7
              Exercise: Practicing Empathy   19

CHAPTER TWO   **The Revolutionary Marriage**   21
              Exercise: Can Open Monogamy Work for Us?   37

CHAPTER THREE **New Models of Monogamy**   39

CHAPTER FOUR **How Do We Start?**   63
              Exercise: Communicating with Empathy   67
              Exercise: Fantasy Scale   78
              Exercise: 3 Ps of Consent   88

CHAPTER FIVE **Navigating Different Needs**   91
              Exercise: Talk and Play   98
              Exercise: Time, Attention, Affection, Sex   105

CHAPTER SIX   **A Promise You Can Keep**   111
              Exercise: Sharing Redlines as Stories   120
              Exercise: Pre-Venting   125

CHAPTER SEVEN **Creating Your Open
              Monogamy Agreement**   127
              Exercise: Finding Your Place on
              the Monogamy Continuum   141

CHAPTER EIGHT **What If It Doesn't Work?**   151
              Exercise: When Your Partner Has Had an Affair   159

CHAPTER NINE   **Aligning with Your True Values**   171

Exercise: Discerning Your Values   179

Exercise: Sibling Triggers   185

Exercise: Sexual Values   187

CONCLUSION   **The Future of Marriage**   195

ACKNOWLEDGEMENTS   201

APPENDIX   **The *Open Monogamy* Interview Structure**   203

GLOSSARY   205

NOTES   209

ABOUT THE AUTHOR   215

NOTE TO READERS

This book applies to all couples and individuals—heterosexual and LGBTQIA+— and to all races and cultures. It is written referring to the pronouns he/she and they. All references to male/female or men/women should be taken with the intent to describe the people interviewed or described as referenced, yet each scenario should be applied to your own personal situation as it fits, in as much as you can take what is said here and make it useful to your own life.

Open Monogamy is inclusive by nature. There is no intent here to harm or leave out any group, gender, orientation, race, or economic class. That said, privilege, inequity, and exclusion show up here just as they do in the overall culture. Also inherent in this book is the idea of couple privilege. Couple privilege means that the couple has more privileges in our society than the single individual. This is not argued for or against, but rather acknowledged as our predominant cultural model. I have used the term marriage to describe a couple who considers themselves *primary partners*. The couple may or may not be living together or legally married.

This is a book about partnership and expanding the definition of relationship. It is intended as a guide for two people who are committed and want to open their relationship to other people, on some level, in some way. In *open monogamy*, the primary relationship comes first. This arrangement is only one point on the *monogamy continuum*. Whether you decide to keep your partnership closed or find yourselves embracing relationship anarchy, you will find the tools here to do it together. Take what works and leave the rest.

Please take all of the content of this book in the spirit it is intended, to help, to support, and to send love to all who need it.

The Relationship of Your Dreams

"You must love in such a way that
the person you love feels free."

THICH NHAT HANH

What if you could have everything you wanted in a relationship? What is the marriage of your dreams? Does it include love, passion, and openness, without dishonesty or indiscretion? If you could be madly in love with your spouse *and* explore outside relationships, would you do it?

If you could stay together in a comforting, warm, connected, and attached partnership without jealousy or fear and still explore sex outside your marriage, would you want to do that, and would you want your partner to explore those options?

What if you had the sex life of your dreams, sharing your desires and fantasies honestly with your partner, opening up in the most vulnerable way about the things you need and want and the things that turn you on? Could you share your erotic life with others?

What else would you include in the relationship of your dreams? What would you add if you could have it all? How far are you from that ideal? Does the possibility of having everything you want feel realistic or more like a dream? Are these your relationship goals? Are they attainable?

Why can't you have all of these things? What is the belief system you have that might be holding you back? Are you afraid that if you ask for what you need, your partner will be angry, fearful, turn away from you, reject you? Maybe they'll feel jealous or hurt. Perhaps there will be tears or arguments.

If you want a more open monogamy but you stifle that desire, don't tell your partner, and keep it to yourself, what will happen? Is that a better choice? Is it a better choice to stay locked into a marriage that makes you feel trapped, unhappy, or stifled?

What if you could have everything you want, and more?

Humans are unique, diverse, and distinctive. We don't all want the same thing. What a boring life we would all lead if we did. There are some things, however, that all of us want. We want to be heard, validated, and understood in a relationship. We want our relationships free from conflict. Not only do we want to avoid conflict with our partner, but we want to avoid our own internal moral conflict that comes from shame, guilt, and the pressure of doing what we think is wrong. We want freedom and security at the same time. We struggle perpetually for safety and for adventure, for exploration and for comfort. These conflicting desires are common to us all.

In many relationships there is what I call a "**monogamy gap**." Couples disagree on the level of openness in their monogamy. This may be caused by a lack of communication, lack of experience, or simply lack of trying. The monogamy gap can lead to conflict, resentment, and for some couples, ultimately separation. Before you get to the catastrophic step of ending your relationship, it's worth it to talk things through to see what kind of changes you can make to your lives. When done right, open monogamy can work. It may be worth it for you to take some chances, rather than ending your relationship for good.

Open monogamy is a form of relationship based on love, commitment, and a desire for honesty and transparency. People in open monogamy relationships value their partners' feelings and have a desire for freedom. They want connection and they sense that their committed partnership could contain more joy, more excitement. They are not held down by their monogamy, but rather, woken up by it. It helps them to expand and grow as individuals as well as partners. They support each other in exploring their needs and desires. They work through the fears and insecurities that naturally come up in any relationship and minimize them when they become conflicts.

John and Julie Gottman, researchers and couples therapists, studied thirty couples for three years in their Love Lab, an apartment laboratory where they watched couples' interactions on video cameras.[1] They found in their research that it is not the amount of conflict that makes for a successful couple, but the attempts to repair the conflict. They found that couples who were successful at repairing were "emotional, vulnerable, and . . . understanding" and validated one another's feelings.

The most powerful conversations began gently, and each partner took responsibility for their part of the problem, working collaboratively. They paid attention when the other had something to say and listened when their partner was upset. This may seem obvious to some—that having a healthy relationship takes communication and listening, validation and responsibility —but if you've ever been married, you know it's harder than it appears.

In an open monogamy, the agreement is not based solely on the desires of one partner. Contrary to the idea that a happy marriage is a well-negotiated quid pro quo arrangement, couples do better when their agreement is based on mutual self-interest. Open monogamy is not the continuation of an affair, nor is it the negotiation of sex outside the relationship in a way that feels threatening or unsafe to the other partner. Open monogamy starts with curiosity, conversations, and a discourse on personal boundaries. The work of making what was implicit explicit is less about having lots of sex parties and more about creating intimacy and expanding the love you can experience, together.

Monogamy is a legal term. It means being married to one person, versus *polygamy*, which means being married to more than one person at a time. We often use the term monogamy interchangeably with *fidelity*, which means being committed to having sex with only one person in a relationship at a time. This is the *traditional* form of monogamy agreement, the explicit promise to have sex with only your partner, until death do you part. *Classical monogamy* has been around for a long time. It is the idea that you wait until marriage to have sex, so that both partners are virgins until their wedding night. They then partner for life, with each being the other's only sexual partner. While this rarely worked out, with infidelity rampant and implicit for centuries, it has been the default in many civilizations.

What is more common in Western society today is *serial monogamy*, where couples are married or partnered with one person and have sex with only that person until the relationship ends. At that time, they meet someone else and commit to be monogamous with them, until that ends and the cycle is repeated.

Open relationships are defined as any type of partnership where rules about monogamy are more fluid. There is less exclusivity and options for sex with people outside the relationship. Swinging, the common name for sexual adventures with other couples, falls into this category, as does polyamory. *Polyamory* encompasses a broader approach, one that includes close emotional, romantic, and sexual relationships outside of the primary partnership. There are many different types and subtypes of open relationships within these categories that we will discuss later in the book.

Some level of nonconformity is inherent in all of us; we want to be independent while at the same time honoring our promises. *Open monogamy* is a way to structure our most intimate relationships in order to balance that search for both commitment and autonomy. Open monogamy simply means being committed, dedicated, loyal, and devoted to one partner while having a consensual understanding to be with other people in some way that's agreeable to you both. Each open monogamy agreement is unique. Couples may agree to be totally closed and traditionally monogamous and at other times wide open. One partner may be open while the other partner may be exclusive. There is no wrong way to have an open monogamy agreement. By its nature, it is workable if it is acceptable to both partners and is open, honest, intentional, and consensual. Some people call this consensual nonmonogamy, others call it ethical nonmonogamy. Some call it being *monogamish*, in an open relationship, or new monogamy. All of these names are creative ways to define being in a flexible, committed partnership with an open relationship agreement.

This book will help you create a uniquely meaningful relationship, one that is accessible, flexible, and fulfilling. Starting with your very first conversation about opening your monogamous relationship, this book explores how to create new boundaries, how to welcome in new partners, how to find balance and excitement, how to change the agreement when things are not working, how and when to be more fluid and flexible, and how to create a vision of the future.

As we as a society move away from traditional monogamy we gravitate toward a more open form of partnership, one with a variety of self-defined limitations, which we can rethink and redefine again. The confines of monogamy can be restrictive, or they can be the platform from which we jump into the unknown, holding the hand of our partner.

INTERVIEWS

The people and the stories you will read here are real. These are all genuine people who shared their authentic journeys with me for the purposes of helping you, the reader. I have changed their names and their identities in order to protect their privacy.

I asked each interviewee a series of questions, which you'll find on page 203. All of the interviewees volunteered more information than I asked for and seemed genuinely interested in sharing information about their relationships.

Some of the stories are taken directly from my psychotherapy sessions. These couples are self-selected, and their names and identities have been changed to protect their privacy. They have successfully navigated the world of open relationships and have struggled with the process. They have fought, doubted, and argued. They have healed from their mistakes and created better boundaries using communication and patience.[2]

In order to understand open and expanded monogamy it's important to look at all sides and all possibilities. As people, we are multifaceted. Like diamonds, we can shine on one side and be hidden in the dark—dusty and cracked—on the other. The stories I will share with you here show the varied faces of humanity in all of its shining beauty.

What you will not find in this book is an argument for or against monogamy. You will not find evidence to show your spouse to prove that you are, indeed, a nonmonogamous mammal, nor research findings to drive you inevitably toward a consensually monogamous relationship. I personally have no investment in your relationship structure. I would like, however, to help you find a way to experience love.

Love can be expressed in a variety of ways. In fact, there are so many ways that it would be unfair of me to say that this book covers them all. But open monogamy is one way to express your love without the restrictions of shame or guilt you may have experienced in the past; it may provide new ways to think about traditional marriage. I have also included many tools in this book to help you create a new open monogamy agreement that might work for you and your partner.

This book will lead you through the steps to opening your monogamy. You may be unsure if this is for you. You may not be ready. You and your partner might not be on the same page. You could be in very different places with your philosophies about open relationships. "Open" means different things to different people. This book will show you how to decide what you want and how to communicate with your partner. I hope it can help you both find the path toward a happy life.

CHAPTER ONE

Expanding Your Love

Marriage is not a guarantee of monogamy. The vow you make at the altar or under the chuppah is a vital promise. Contrary to popular opinion, it is not a guarantee of forever.

A wedding is a celebration. The wedding vow you make on the day you celebrate your marriage is a promise, and that vow should be real, for sure, but a one-time vow on one special day is not going to last a lifetime. A one-time promise is not a guarantee of monogamy or sexual fidelity. It doesn't cover all of the changes you will go through in a shared lifetime—all the stressors, the arguments, the illnesses, the children, the financial troubles, and the difficulties of real-life are part of the natural ups and downs of a relationship. To weather these changes, you need something more. You need an everyday vow.

Your wedding vow is not the ultimate promise. It takes something more to make a marriage work. It takes a constant pledge to preserve, sustain, maintain, and/or uphold your obligation to each other.

Monogamy is a decision you make *every day*; the choice to be monogamous is always on your terms. Some days are harder than others, which is why *you should adjust your monogamy to fit your relationship. You don't have to adjust your relationship to fit your monogamy. Adjusting your monogamy to fit your life is more practical and more realistic.*

An oath, pledge, promise, or vow you make to another person is something you will have to revisit over and over. You will have to adjust your meaning of open monogamy as you grow so that the agreement fits your lifestyle and needs.

Instead of examining your partner to see how they do or don't meet your ideal vision, instead of blaming them for why you can't remain monogamous or keep your vow, you can instead commit to adjusting your monogamy agreement every day of your lives. Examine together how your agreement fits your lives. **If it's not working, change the agreement. Don't change your partner.** *You don't have to change your partner if you are both willing to change the arrangement.*

DO IT YOUR WAY

There are many ways to live and love and no simple guidelines for living in our complex world. Each one of us and every one of our emotional experiences are unique. Everyone alive has a distinct style of expressing love in a relationship, and these feelings can change throughout a lifetime. Romantic love is unique in this way.

Deciding to be in a relationship is the first step. After that, there's usually a lot of flailing around, taking chances, and heartbreak. It's a struggle to get it right.

For whatever reason, the two of you have come together to love each other, and you're doing it. You're finding your way. But you sense there could be more, a more significant kind of love, a love that expresses and encompasses more delight with the world, and more joy. You want a relationship that embraces the whole experience of love.

What makes your particular relationship exceptional is that no one's ever done it before. There's never been a pair like the two of you in the history of the universe. All the books, podcasts, and online advice columnists tell you to do it this way or that way. They ask you to call it one thing or another. Some of what you read or hear works for you, but other parts don't apply. You are looking for a clear path, a direction, a way to keep the parts of your relationship that are good but make it more expansive.

The two of you are special. You don't want to mess this up. You want your relationship to work. You want to love each other with fairness and integrity because that's what you signed up for and honesty aligns with your shared values. You want to know how to stick to those values and be honest about what you want without hurting each other. But you also want more.

You want answers.

The bad news? There is no one right way to do this. The good news? You can have anything you want. I am going to tell you how.

MONOGAMY AS A VERB

Many people, like you, are finding that traditional monogamy no longer encompasses the myriad of ways there are to love. There can be hurt and confusion when you try to fit into a *closed monogamy agreement*, an agreement where sexual and emotional connection stays between two specified partners. It can feel restrictive and at times punitive and doesn't encompass the broader vision of your best life. You sense that if you could love the way you want, life would feel more spacious. You wouldn't have to try to fit into a life that doesn't makes sense for you.

By definition, open monogamy is open to interpretation, your interpretation. It starts with being vulnerable with each other; open to the conversation and a new definition that's limited only by your imagination.

Open monogamy means you have a primary partner with whom you also have a flexible relationship agreement. This agreement can include emotional, romantic, and open sexual behaviors with other people. Open monogamy is a way to structure your commitment. You can have a little structure or lots of rules, it's totally up to you.

> Open monogamy means you have a primary partner with whom you also have a flexible relationship agreement. You can have little structure or lots of rules, it's totally up to you.

People of all ages and backgrounds are moving away from traditional monogamy and gravitating toward more open partnerships, ones with a variety of definitions. This new form of monogamy is flexible and unique to each couple. It is an agreement that works for your life.

From the first conversation, open monogamy is about creating new and expanded boundaries. It means changing your relationship agreement to make things better and then shifting again when things are not working. Open monogamy is a fluid and flexible form of monogamy. It could mean finding more pleasure and excitement together, in private, or it could mean welcoming in new partners. Couples who practice open monogamy co-create a vision of their ideal future and continuously redefine it.

Many couples who consider themselves primary partners see their relationship as essential to their lives. Styles vary, and the way they create their monogamy can vary from year to year or even day-to-day.

You can modify it to work in any way that is comfortable for the two of you. Monogamy is not something you do in your head; it's something you do together. *You can't be monogamous alone.* It takes two people to be monogamous. Therefore, you have to agree on the meaning of monogamy between you.

Monogamy is not something you choose once, it's something you create over and over, revisiting its definition regularly.

EXPANDING THE LOVE

You love your partner. Your desire for a more flexible monogamy agreement has nothing to do with what's missing or lacking in *them*. You may be delighted to be together and still want to expand on what you already have, making what's right even better.

That's the funny thing about love. It expands, it doesn't contract. When you love someone, you want to share more of yourself with them, bringing more of who you are into the relationship. You can envision something big for yourself and your relationship; the two of you, side by side, living your biggest and best life, sharing the potential of a flexible and fluid relationship.

Opening yourself to your partner in a real, deep, and meaningful way is the core of open monogamy. Pushing into the potential of what your relationship could be can also be scary. Growth is frightening. Being in open or expanded monogamy is a radical way to love someone. It's not for everyone.

This decision should be mutual. It should come from a place of love, not from a place of confusion or frustration. Don't do this because something is going wrong or things are going poorly at home. (NOTE: If you aren't doing well as a couple, try starting with the empathy exercises at the end of this chapter and in chapter 4. Just because you are in conflict doesn't mean you cannot work it out. For serious conflicts, find a counselor that understands your issues and resolve the more serious problems before you come back to expanding your monogamy.)

Expanding your monogamy isn't necessarily a sign that your love isn't working. It could mean the opposite. Adding to your relationship or expanding it can be a way to express more respect for each other.

Creating an open monogamy agreement can be an expression of love that's unique and exclusive to the two of you *and* whomever you choose to invite into that love. For some, an open agreement is a way to celebrate the good fortune in having found one another, and a way to spread the blessing.

Giving someone space to be the person they want to be can be the most loving thing you can do in a relationship. It doesn't mean detaching from them or being emotionally distant. It is a way of showing love that allows for differentiation, allowing each of you to be separate people and honoring the independent experience, while still staying attached.

Giving a partner freedom *within* the relationship encourages them to grow and expand into the person they want to be. It lets them know that they can stretch into the areas they want to explore and grow as an individual, which ultimately gives them more to bring to the relationship. Giving your partner freedom shows them that they can be curious, that their interest in the world is not a bad thing, and that you can accept their inquisitiveness. This freedom allows for more risks and exploration. In a grown-up relationship, this can be a healthier way to relate as adults.

Letting go of fear and giving your partner space and freedom implies confidence in them and in oneself as well as in the relationship. The ability to relate to each other as whole people with separate experiences in life is important in order to avoid feeling threatened by the other's personal growth.

If you have found love, you have been lucky. You may want to share that luck. If you have built a solid foundation together, you can now expand your relationship to include other people. You have enough to go around.

Welcome to the beginning of discovering more of yourself, embracing more of your significant other, and enlarging the relationship.

THE BRIDGE

Monogamy is like a bridge. You work on your side of the bridge by thinking clearly about what you want, what works for you, and continuously examining your part in the relationship. Your partner does the same on their side of the bridge. These ends hold up the whole structure. Continually reinforcing the endpoints makes them durable enough to endure the intense lateral pressure of the road between them. You are each responsible for building the strength of your end of the bridge.

Only when your ends are healthy can you reach across the arch, connect, and define the bridge's structure. When you stretch and extend toward the other, you create the road. Until then, you are only in a relationship with yourself, thinking you are together in your head. It takes more than making promises to the other person. Just saying the words does not a relationship make. Vows have no meaning if you have not created them using words that have importance to you personally, and you have not agreed on them as a couple. The words should be alive, vibrant, and ever-changing.

Once you reach out and meet on the bridge, you are ready to talk about what you both want. You bring your strengths, fears, and experiences, and as two, whole, differentiated people, you are better prepared to commit to the relationship. When you arrive on the bridge, you can decide what you want and what is right for the two of you.

If you decide you want something other than a traditional monogamous partnership, you will have the tools, after reading this book, to create your new monogamy agreement. It will be unique to your needs, flexible and fluid, and able to change as you grow as a couple. You can create anything you want. You are each responsible for holding up your side of the bridge and are accountable for how you show up on the road to meet your partner. No one else can be accountable to your agreement, only the two of you. No one else is at fault if it goes wrong, and only the two of you are liable if you make mistakes.

It is all totally up to you. Make this the start of the new road that leads to your new relationship.

HOW DO WE DO THIS?

A successful open monogamy agreement works when it expands the love you have for each other. By working through this book, you will decide what kind of open agreement will enhance your lives. You are going to create something that will help you grow into better people. You will be asked to look at your own views on monogamy and relationships and decide if open monogamy is for you and what kind might work in your ideal relationship and suit you best. This is the foundation for a relationship with your partner, and later, potentially, multiple partners. Then you will learn the skills to approach your partner, ask for what you want, and create the relationship of your dreams. You will learn how to manage it all and how to shut it down when it's not working.

An open monogamy agreement shouldn't contract things between you. It won't make you feel afraid, angry, coerced, or upset. When you do feel those feelings, you will need to know how to talk with your partner and resolve things right away.

If you are like most of my clients, you trust each other enough to know that love like yours is worth keeping. Because your relationship is strong, it can take some stretching. If you are careful and do this consciously, the mindful growth of your relationship is not going to separate you; it's going to make you closer.

Can Open Monogamy Work for You?

In my thirty-plus years as a therapist seeing couples struggle to stay true to their agreements or true to each other, I can tell you that open monogamy is not for everyone. To determine if open monogamy could work for you, start by asking yourself the following:

Am I emotionally flexible?

Can I reach out for support when I need it?

Can I be fair?

Do I play well with others?

Can I share?

Can I have real conversations with my partner?

Am I patient?

Can I let go of possessiveness?

Do I handle jealousy well?

Can I be empathetic?

How did you answer these questions? Do your answers indicate places that need your attention? These are all relationship proficiencies and areas where you can learn to improve. These are places that show you where you need to do personal work, your areas of self-development, and the foundation of your side of the bridge. They are skills that will help you in any relationship, and you will want to be proficient in these if you are going to open your marriage. But you don't have to be perfect in any of these areas; they are emotional skills you'll need to work at over a lifetime.

These questions are designed to bring attention to areas that you might want to look at about before you take the plunge. They are relationship skills that matter in all contexts and are important to develop in yourself in order to feel satisfied and emotionally competent as an adult.

LAURA AND JOHN

Laura and John have been together for five years. Laura is an attorney and John works in construction. They came to therapy to explore opening their monogamy.

When Laura was growing up, her mother wouldn't let her out of her sight. Laura's father had died in a tragic car accident when she was young. Her mother never got over her father's death. Her mother followed her around as a toddler and was by her side well into her teens. She wouldn't let Laura play sports because she was afraid she would get hurt. She wouldn't let her drive. When it was time, she discouraged Laura from going to college out of state, pleading with her to stay close to home.

Laura felt her mother stifled her curiosity and natural wonder about the world. Her mother's anxiety over her safety made her hold too tight to Laura and smothered Laura's desire for exploration. Laura felt she never had freedom to be herself. She craved it now.

In their marriage, John was encouraging of Laura. He wanted her to go out and explore and grow. He pushed her to go to law school, telling her she was smart and she needed to follow her dreams. She was grateful and yet she felt guilty. She wanted more.

In therapy, Laura said they had a dilemma; she had a desire for freedom and yet she had an overwhelming feeling of responsibility to John and their marriage. Laura felt she couldn't balance these two things and needed help.

Laura had met someone, a man, and they had grown close. She started traveling for work and spending time with him. In the session, Laura confessed to John, "I think I might be attracted to this person and I am afraid we might be more than just friends. Can we talk about this?"

John said yes, he was open to having the conversation. Laura was concerned that John would be like her mother, that he would hold her too close, keep her home, and constrict her movements. She felt she was unable to talk to John openly without having a therapist guide the dialogue. She was afraid John would feel threatened by her desire to meet new people and maybe even to open up their marriage.

In fact, John felt supportive of her feelings. He said he was glad that she had been honest with him. He said, "I want you to grow. I want you to expand as a person. I don't feel threatened in that way. I want you to be happy. Thank you for not keeping this a secret."

Laura was astonished, and their conversations in therapy continued. Both shared their concerns, their fears, and their excitement about where this could take them, both together and separately.

We will get back to more of Laura and John's story later in the book. But their story is not unprecedented. It's estimated that 4 to 5 percent of people (about three million couples) in the United States today are in a consensually nonmonogamous relationship.[1] These numbers include married and dedicated partners who have outside sexual and emotional contact with other people. (If 4 to 5 percent of Americans don't seem like a lot of people, keep in mind 4.5 percent of the population identify as LGBTQIA+.)[2] The central tenet of a consensually nonmonogamous relationship is that both partners know about the external connections. Everything is consensual, and the rules and boundaries and feelings are transparent. In most cases, both of the partners can participate in outside relationships. The relationships may be private or shared. *Consensual nonmonogamy* can mean anything the partners decide it should mean.

All of these relationships, no matter what they look like, happen after discussion, agreement, and consent. The foundation of these essential ingredients is empathy.

EMPATHY

Love doesn't automatically imply agreement. You can love your partner and have very different opinions about life. You are separate people, you come from different backgrounds and have varying viewpoints. You may even argue. It doesn't matter if you agree on everything; you are each distinctive people with original ideas about life. Most couples disagree. Love means being able to empathize with your partner, not to concur on everything.

What is empathy and why is it important? What prevents it and how do we achieve it in a relationship?

Empathy is a state of relational safety and connection that allows for exploration and curiosity about your partner.

Empathy is a state of relational safety and connection that allows for exploration and curiosity about your partner. Empathy means being curious about what it's like to be the other person. Empathy is trying to understand how the other person experiences life, why they want certain things, their fantasies, desires, and emotions—all of which may be different from your own. You don't have to have the same feelings or fantasies or desires or emotions. Your partner's experience is most likely distinctive from yours. The goal is not to feel the same or reach the same conclusions about things in life. But if you love someone, you will try to empathize with them.

Why Be Empathetic?

Empathy prevents the splitting off of your needs from the relationship. When you feel your partner is empathetic with you, you are more likely to bring your feelings, needs, and desires to them. Even if they can't meet all of your needs, if you know they will try and understand them, you are more likely to communicate and share with your partner instead of hiding or lying about what you feel and think.

If you feel your partner consistently disagrees with your feelings or shuts you down, you will eventually feel unheard. Talking about being in an open relationship, especially at first, can be challenging. Learning empathy is important for these conversations.

Empathy leads to improved communication and emotional generosity. If you feel your partner is trying to be empathetic, if they validate your experience, they don't need to agree with everything you say. It won't matter if they have their own opinion or if it differs from yours. Each of you is entitled to your view of the world. If you feel that your viewpoint is honored, you will feel connected and understood even if you disagree about whose opinion is right.

When you feel heard in this way, when your partner tries to empathize with you—even if they don't agree with you—it lends comfort to the relationship. You are more likely to be yourself, take risks, and ask for what you want. It doesn't mean you are going to get what you want, but an empathetic, compassionate relationship can lead to more open communication. This is key to a better open marriage.

If you feel comfortable in your relationship, if you know your partner empathizes with what you feel, you will feel more comfortable asking for what you want. *What would you ask for if you felt safe asking for what you want?*

What Prevents Empathy?

- Fear of our curiosity and fantasies
- Fear that your partner will act out your fantasies before you are ready
- Fear of being judged
- Fear of the loss of connection
- Projection of our fears onto our partner

What Is the Result of Empathy?

- Intimacy and connection
- Being open
- Being giving
- Being willing to change

Practicing Empathy

How can you begin to communicate your emotional needs to your partner? The following exercise will help you develop empathy for your partner. Fill out the rest of these sentence stems in a journal:

One thing that *you* do that makes *me* feel loved:

I appreciate this because:

One thing *I* can do to make *you* feel more loved:

I know you like this because:

One thing I know you want more of in our relationship:

That makes sense to me because:

I would like to make your life easier by:

I'd like to do this because I think you need more:

As you are thinking about your answers, what feelings come up? Can you share this with your partner? Why or why not? If not, don't worry. You'll find another exercise in empathy later in the book.

ↄ

CHAPTER TWO

The Revolutionary Marriage

Marriage today is optional. This is a relatively new concept. For women, the choice to be married, to marry later, or even to keep one's name, is due in part to the hard-earned battles of the feminist movement. Over the past one hundred years freedoms claimed by women have reformed the institution of marriage.

In the past, marriage was a legal contract meant to control women and their reproduction. In a patriarchal society, it was necessary to have a system that would guarantee a man's paternity and control procreation.[1] A husband who wanted to pass down property to his heirs wanted to be sure his children belonged solely to him. Marriage was about ownership, and the wife was property, controlled by her husband. Forced to give up her name, she lost her freedom and her identity in exchange for shared ownership and security.

In 1960, the first oral contraceptive was approved by the Food and Drug Administration, but it wasn't until 1965 that the Supreme Court gave married women the right to use birth control. Even then, women in twenty-six states did not have access to the pill. In 1972, birth control pills were legalized for all married and unmarried women.[2]

With birth control legal and accessible, women no longer had to worry about unwanted pregnancies. Women were more in control of their bodies and had more say in when and with whom they would be sexual.

In the 1960s and 1970s, the boundaries and values changed around sex. The sexual revolution had begun. Women found their power in sex and couples began to explore relationships in new ways. The book *Open Marriage* by George and Nena O'Neill came out in 1972 and was on the

New York Times best seller list for forty weeks.[3] It was translated into fourteen languages and sold more than thirty-five million copies.

Open Marriage was a book about free love, a primer on how to be equal in a partnership, including a guide to sharing childcare responsibilities. It also included thoughts about opening the relationship to outside sexual partners. Although there were only a few lines in the book about opening up sexually, including, "Sexual fidelity is the false god of closed marriage,"[4] these ideas lit a fire in a society that was looking for more leeway in relationships.

The book supported equal rights for women, inside of the marriage. But it was still hard for women to get out of an unhappy marriage. Domestic violence, neglectful husbands, or just bad matches were irrelevant. With the burden of childcare and unequal pay, it wasn't easy for a woman to leave. Many women stayed married, even if their husband cheated or abused them.

In 1973, women were granted the right to a no-fault divorce and no longer had to feel trapped if they wanted out. When they could receive alimony and child support, it made it possible to get divorced and still have the financial resources to move on as a single person. With that support, they could be independent and keep their children. They no longer needed to stay in ill-fated marriages.

THE STATE OF MARRIAGE TODAY

In 2020, during the COVID-19 pandemic, divorce rates rose by 25 percent in China after the three months of sheltering-in-place order was lifted. This is similar to 2003, when one year after the SARS-CoV outbreak, the divorce rate in Hong Kong was 21 percent higher than the year prior.[5]

According to the Chief Justice and President of the Supreme People's Court Zhou Qiang at Tsinghua University in China, it is the woman, 74 percent of the time, who initiates the divorce. The women who had quarantined with their husbands left and left permanently. After the long stretch of forced isolation and the stress of an unhappy relationship, they decided that they no longer wanted to be married.

These decisions are never easy. Separation and divorce are always tricky, which may be why more people are deciding not to marry at all or to marry later. More adults are living together and don't plan on ever marrying, according to a 2019 Pew Research Center survey.[6]

In addition, as of 2019, more adults—ages 18 to 44—have lived with an unmarried partner (59 percent) than have ever been married (50 percent), according to a Pew Research Center analysis of the National Survey of Family Growth.

However, the survey found that married adults are more satisfied with their relationship and more trusting of their partners than those who just live together. Spouses trust their partner; they believe they won't cheat and trust them to tell the truth and act in their best interest. Married couples are more satisfied with their relationships (58 percent) and say things are going well, compared to couples living together, who say that 41 percent of the time.

Yet most people, 78 percent, say it's acceptable to live together without getting married.[7] We don't have to marry someone to have sex or to have a child or to get a mortgage or to legitimize our union. The commitment to the contract of marriage is not mandatory. Marriage is a choice both men and women make purely out of a desire for a romantic ideal. This relationship promise binds them to another person out of noncompulsory, idealistic tradition. And love.

A couple chooses to be together because they see a future with one another, and whether implicit or explicit, the rules of their monogamy contract apply—until they don't. Their agreement around sexual fidelity encompasses a shared life; it is supposed to be a lifetime commitment.

In some ways, we are still operating under old marriage rules. Many women still take their husband's last names, all inheritance passes through the male line, and in many cases, when a wife divorces her husband, she loses her financial stability. Women are less secure in their careers because of the institutional fear that women will leave their job to have children, and women are more often primarily responsible for childcare.

But, marriage as it stands now is no longer based on the standards of monogamy created several hundred years ago. With the high rates of divorce and even higher rates of infidelity, couples seem to be struggling with these old patriarchal definitions of marriage and monogamy appears to be morphing into something new. These changes to the meaning of marriage reflect an underlying conflict around equality and a desire to create something that better reflects our current lifestyle, something more egalitarian. This conflict means growth is trying to happen. Changes are happening, but there are still barriers.

Monogamy as Morality

Traditional marriage may be outdated, but we still believe monogamy to be synonymous with morality. Morality has been more of a religious concept than a social value, thrust upon us during an age of Christianity when the church established a patriarchal hierarchy to ensure the validity of male inheritance. A patriarchal lineage ensured the passing down of sheep and other property. It also restricted female sexuality. In a recent Gallup poll people said that cheating on a spouse was morally the worst of all behaviors. When asked what they thought of monogamy, Americans said an affair is worse than suicide and gambling. And 60 percent said infidelity was worse than human cloning.[8]

Monogamy, therefore, is often a reflection of character, a sign of a good or bad person, even though its true definition simply means being married to one person. We use the term monogamy as a moral imperative, a judgment meant to imply sexual exclusivity.

As baby boomers age and millennials grow up and make their own marital decisions, we are entering a new era. It seems we still want some kind of monogamy, but we can be freer with its definition. A desire for both freedom and connection, for safety and adventure, and a love that comes with a guarantee of aliveness is the new ideal. We increasingly seek to be an individual and pursue our own needs while remaining in committed relationship to another.

In 2016, a government study found that many couples prefer a more nuanced, nonmonogamous relationship to traditionally monogamous marriage. When asked about their "ideal" relationship, only 61 percent of all adults chose "0, or completely monogamous," and even fewer—51 percent—of Americans age 18 to 30 did.[9]

These are fundamental changes in how we see marriage, a revolution in monogamy, a paradigm shift in the way we partner. It is a way to branch out from a strictly closed form of monogamy and explore a new definition of romantic partnership. The couples in my therapy office are defining their morality and operating traditional marriages in a whole new way.

This is part of a larger cultural trend. We no longer define marriage as an agreement between a man and a woman. The DOMA, or Defense of Marriage Act, was struck down in much of the United States. This means it is legal for two men, two women, or two gender diverse people of any identification to marry legally. The church is much less involved in marriage because fewer people are religious. Only 22 percent of weddings took place at religious institutions in 2017.[10] That's down from 41 percent in 2009. More people choose to have their ceremony on a beach or in a barn, in a field or in a hall. Marriage is no longer defined by the church or by gender or sexual identity, but by love and the desire to commit.

Meanwhile, the government is in our bedrooms more than they have been in decades. The increasing desire to create personalized versions of marriage could be a reaction to that intrusion. When religion or government tells us what, who, and how to love, it is called repression. When couples react and push back, demanding more personal freedoms, it portends the beginning of a new era, a new level of self-determination. We may find what works in a way we have never experienced before.

There is so much more to come.

Marriage, one hundred years ago, was:
- Defined by organized religion
- Between two people—one male and one female
- A legally sanctioned religious ritual
- A civil union to one person, forever
- A contract which bound you to physical proximity
- A commitment to sexual fidelity
- A legal contract in which men took ownership of any shared property

Then, marriage morphed into something different:
- You don't have to get married in or by the church
- Marriage is not limited to heterosexuals
- Marriage is no longer a contract for life

- You can marry many times in a lifetime
- Many people have a long-distance marriage
- Divorce is legal, and most states are
  community property states
- You can be married and have multiple partners

IT TAKES A REVOLUTION

Merriam-Webster's Collegiate Dictionary defines revolution as "a sudden, radical, or complete change."[11]

A cultural revolution happens when a cultural norm no longer works for the people who are repressed. There is a need to evolve, to change, and make a radical change. In the 1960s and 1970s, a counterculture formed, one that attempted to make ineffective or restrain or neutralize the ill effects of the current culture, which repressed women and marginalized outsiders. By creating an opposing force, people rose. They took action, some with protests, some in the courtroom, and some by subtle influence. Revolution happens when there is a push for change, when one paradigm is substituted for another, when a movement affects fundamental shifts of belief. Revolutionary periods alter the way we think about or visualize our world, and change to the paradigm is permanent.

If we also think about a revolution as "the time taken by a celestial body to make a complete round in its orbit," it is an interesting metaphor for this new revolution in monogamy. The completion of a rotation—or revolution—is a measure in time; it is a progressive motion, and eventually, that motion returns to its initial position, but it is changed forever by its journey. The revolution creates something altogether different and the experience of resistance helps the culture shift and grow into something that's better for everyone.

In the section on "Honest Communication, Productive Fighting and Equality" in the book *Open Marriage*, the authors say that sex outside the marriage could make marriage "a still deeper, richer, more vital experience." Later they insisted that this was misinterpreted. They said the "open" in the title referred more to sharing and open communication, not specifically sex with other people.

In later interviews, the authors were more neutral about the "open" part of an open marriage, "We are not recommending outside sex, but we are not saying that it should be avoided, either. The choice is entirely up to you."

In 1977, Nena O'Neill wrote *The Marriage Premise* and went back to a more traditional stance of fidelity in marriage. "The whole area of extramarital sex is touchy," she said in *The New York Times*. "I don't think we ever saw it as a concept for the majority, and certainly, it has not proved to be."[12]

OPEN RELATIONSHIPS

Today, a half-century after *Open Marriage* was published and post-pandemic, we now have new definitions of committed partnerships: open, fluid, polyamorous. These terms all include some kind of base relationship that falls on a continuum of monogamy.

An open relationship means having sexual, emotional, and romantic partnerships with people outside of a primary relationship, with permission. A traditionally closed relationship is exclusive, presumably without outside sexual, emotional, or romantic experiences.

In an open relationship, both partners have an arrangement that is unique to them, but at times, this arrangement needs to be revisited to apply to current circumstances. There is no wrong way to have an open relationship, but it needs to be transparent, honest, intentional, and consensual.

An open relationship means a couple defines their monogamy agreement in a way that allows for outside partners, either when they are together or separately. It can work if both partners are communicative, cooperative, and have a solid foundation of trust. Creating a monogamy agreement with clear rules can help.

Does It Work?

People who value open monogamy say that it allows them to displace unmet needs that can't be met by one person. They credit this benefit alone with increasing relationship satisfaction.

Western culture perpetuates the expectation that one romantic partner should meet all of an individual's needs.[13] But some people argue that today's traditionally monogamous marriages ask too much of one partner.

One partner is expected to fulfill all of the physical, sexual, parental, companionate, financial, and self-actualization needs, which puts too much pressure on one person. Because we expect more from our partners than ever before, and at the same time, invest less time and effort in our relationships than ever before, it's impossible for one person to meet these higher-level needs.[14]

During the pandemic-caused quarantines and lockdowns of 2020 and 2021, we saw more couples than ever realizing that their marriages were either boring or that one partner failed to meet their sexual needs. In fact, 18.2 percent of men and 26.4 percent of women perceived a decrease in sexual desire over the year.[15] Many found that the increase in stress and worry over the pandemic may have contributed to lack of desire, but also noted that the increase in domesticity and responsibility led to decreased interest in their primary partner. We know that sex, pleasure, and desire decrease with domesticity, exhaustion, and parenting responsibilities. It is possible that an increased awareness of the need for multiple partners will continue in order to handle domestic and parenting responsibilities as well as romantic and sexual duties in committed relationships.

Open monogamy could be the answer.

DIVORCE AND INFIDELITY

Divorce is a part of marriage. There is no getting around that fact. Now, when we marry, we no longer assume we will marry for a lifetime. Divorce in this country is so prevalent it would be irrational to think that a bride or groom never think about divorce as a possibility when they say their vows. Divorce rates for first marriages are at 42 to 45 percent, 60 percent for second marriages, and 73 percent for third marriages.[16]

Cheating is one thing that hasn't changed from the bad old days; it's as popular as ever and more accessible. With the high rates of infidelity,[17] marriage is no guarantee of sexual exclusivity. With the ease of online sites like Ashley Madison, the married dating site, which surpassed the seventy million member mark at the end of 2020,[18] it is easier than ever for infidelity to interfere with a marriage. With smartphones in hand, this is the first time in history where you can cheat on your partner while lying in bed next to them.

More couples than ever can recover from infidelity, however. And some can negotiate a more fluid type of monogamy[19] after an affair, opening their relationship to include outside partners or sexual agreements that do not threaten their emotional monogamy. The integrity of the relationship is maintained through emotional commitment, not sexual exclusivity.

Choosing to get married at all seems like a revolutionary decision these days. With the high rates of divorce and even higher incidents of infidelity, the traditional form of marriage, with an expectation of one partner for life, doesn't seem to stick. We continue to get married and try to honor it, but we don't do it well. Studies show that *we break our agreement before we try to change it*. We believe somehow that holding on to the appearance of monogamy is better than changing it to fit our real lives. Instead, we lie and cheat and eventually divorce, instead of modifying our agreement.

> The integrity of the relationship is maintained through emotional commitment, not sexual exclusivity.

Lying and cheating aren't making us happy. It's not the solution for a happier marriage. We don't like to cheat and we don't want to lie to our partner, but we still do it.

When we look at infidelity statistics, the future looks bleak. Is infidelity inevitable when we try to live up to the outdated expectations of a long-term marriage with one person? My experience with hundreds of couples tells me it is at least very likely.

Polyamory

Polyamory is a specific form of open relationship that isn't just about sex with other people. It includes loving relationships, emotional connections that may or may not include both spouses. In polyamorous relationships, there's enough love to go around, and relationships with outside people don't limit the love for one another.

Polyamory comes from the words *poly*, meaning many, and *amor*, meaning love. Polyamorous arrangements vary from couple to couple and within different relationships in a *polycule* or a pod. Couples interested in being polyamorous need to talk about all of the options, particularly when they first decide to try polyam. Choosing how they might structure things from the beginning can prevent problems later on, but the agreement shouldn't be definitive. Everything should be fluid and decided on as things move along.

IS OPEN MONOGAMY A BETTER OPTION?

In studies done on individuals in monogamous relationships and in consensually nonmonogamous relationships, it was found they both have similar levels of passionate love. However, jealousy was lower and trust higher among those in consensually nonmonogamous relationships. It's not clear whether people who are not jealous in general are more attracted to open relationships, or if jealousy levels are lower as a result of being open.

Compared with monogamous people, polyamorous people were significantly more satisfied, more committed, and more trusting of their partners. They also had lower levels of jealous behaviors than their monogamous counterparts. Passionate love was also higher among polyamorous individuals than monogamous individuals.

The studies are interesting, but only in that the researchers guess that it "could indicate that the polyamorous style of relationships—in which both sexual intimacy and emotional intimacy with multiple people are allowed—is particularly effective. If one of the purposes of sex is emotional intimacy, perhaps it is more difficult for an individual to be satisfied in one relationship while attempting to suppress emotional and romantic feelings for others with whom that individual is sexual, as is expected in strictly open relationships or swinging. Another possibility is that polyamorous people are more likely to utilize communication strategies that are effective."[20]

Strictly monogamous couples have a lot to learn here. The supposition is that polyam couples actually are more trusting and less jealous because they communicate more often, they can express their desires without reproach, they are allowed to have their needs met without shame, and they feel heard and validated around those needs. Whether it is easy or not is not the question, and we will discuss this as the book progresses. What seems to be the important takeaway from this study is that an open monogamy is possible and with potentially positive results.

MY OWN REVOLUTIONARY MARRIAGE

My husband and I have been married for many years and we raised our four children together—his two girls and my son and daughter. Our home was in a small town in Connecticut, close enough to my office in downtown New Haven and far enough into the rural suburbs that we had to drive fifteen minutes to buy milk.

It was the second marriage for both of us, and we were committed not only to each other but to all of our children. In our vows we promised that we would love and be there for the kids for life. This commitment kept us going through good times and bad. When I grew frustrated over the years, I would remember the pledge, and it got me through the more challenging years of raising a blended family.

In the early years, we had the luxury of every other weekend to ourselves. Every two weeks, he and I had two glorious days to focus on our intimate grown-up lives. Most of those weekends, we never got out of bed. Our undivorced and remarried friends expressed their envy at our ability to luxuriate in our exciting, uninterrupted time together. As the kids grew, our every other weekend routine faded. We missed our alone time together.

When my youngest daughter left for college, I knew I would move back to the West Coast, where I had been born. My husband agreed it was time for a change. The New England winters were dark and cold, and sunny California called.

Then, life changed. My mother-in-law got sick. My husband went to New Jersey to take care of her. We thought it was a temporary situation. He wanted to be there for her and I agreed.

It's been several years now. We sold our house in Connecticut and I moved to California full time. He is living a bicoastal life, spending time in New Jersey as a companion to his ninety-six-year-old mother. I am living in Los Angeles. I am happy. I am in the sun. But I miss my husband.

We spent many long nights discussing our relationship and how we would manage our monogamy. What would our sex life look like? How would we stay connected? What was intimacy like when our closest exchanges were three thousand miles apart? What was bicoastal life going to be like for the two of us?

Then, the pandemic hit and travel became more difficult. Flying back and forth was risky, given the health factors in our family. The wait for a vaccine was long and unsure.

When we were together in Los Angeles, the days were languorous and lovely, connected and sunny. We did what most people new to California do; we hiked and went to the beach and drove to Joshua Tree. We spent all of our time together because we both worked from home. The virus kept us together, as it did many people in the world. We were lucky. It made us closer, instead of driving us apart.

Then we got vaccinated. He went back to New Jersey and our bicoastal life began again.

LIVING APART TOGETHER

For now, we are still together, still a couple, but are in what I call a living-apart-together (LAT) relationship. LAT relationships are not uncommon these days; fourteen million people in the United States have long-distance relationships.

With the increase in technological advances, online platforms, and interactive sex toys, many couples maintain a LAT relationship across long distances, and some do so even when they are only miles apart.

Many LAT couples are sexually monogamous, while others are only romantically or emotionally exclusive. Other couples take it on a case-by-case basis. Some consider themselves "sex-toy committed," meaning that they can have orgasms with technology, whether together or with others virtually, but never with someone other than their partner in the flesh, in real life. Several porn sites and sex-toy companies have combined forces to integrate movies with teledildonics that make the virtual reality experience feel real to the viewer. They integrate 4D technology with virtual reality headsets for a fully immersive visual experience. When used with a sex toy, it becomes an interactive experience as well. The human element is added by a remote partner who controls the interactions in order to mimic a real sexual encounter. With many people more isolated than ever before, virtual reality robots and artificial intelligence may decrease isolation and be a part of every couple's monogamy conversation.

Other couples negotiate their open monogamy agreement so they can each see other people when they are apart. In this scenario, both partners welcome their spouse's desire for companionship, knowing they can't be there for the other person.

There are many forms of LAT agreements. Some couples date other people while they travel but not in the city where either of them resides. They may decide to remain emotionally faithful and committed to each other but have a *don't ask, don't tell policy*. We will cover all of these arrangements later in the book.

My husband and I have an exceptional marriage and we work hard at staying connected. Our arrangement works for us, for now, but it won't work forever. Some nights are harder than others. One thing I know for sure about our marriage is that it will change. It has changed dramatically so many times over the years that I wonder how I ever thought we could define it as one thing. Defining our monogamy, as I look back, seems like chasing a fish in a pond. The moment we felt it was one thing, everything shifted; we grew, life happened. The most important lesson I have learned over the years as a wife and as a therapist is this: things change.

My Husband's Experience Living Apart Together

I wanted to know how my husband experienced our long-distance relationship so that I could share it here. This is what he wrote:

> Monogamy is a state of mind. It represents a commitment to honor the trust previously established between partners. In the event monogamous partners are unable to be with each other physically for an extended time, it is only natural to feel incomplete and alone.
>
> Technology helps bridge the otherwise empty feeling that comes when you physically are not together. Even so, it never is quite the same. Staring into each other's eyes on a screen will never be a replacement for lying next to them. The screen doesn't transmit a breath. You can't reach out and touch their skin or gently bite their lip.
>
> Distant relationships have a way of filtering out all the meaningless side issues and putting the focus on why you became a couple in the first place. It's a distillation process that yields love. And once you see the purity of love, then the relationship's true essence prevails, which, in turn, strengthens the desire to preserve the monogamous agreement.

While it's true all relationships have high and low points, a protracted distance relationship will often alter the ups and downs. It is further complicated when they are in different time zones. The good times never feel as good as when you're physically together. However, the lows can create a more profound feeling of despair that can challenge the underlying bond.

The alone times brings a different element of individualism, a broader sense of independence blended with a much different understanding of interdependent commitment. When a monogamous partner lives with you, there's the expectation you will see them that day. Your actions are, in part, affected by your knowing you'll see them, touch them, hug them, and kiss them sometime that day. It contributes to the shape of your daily workflow, both focused and free flow. It alters your conscious decisions while shaping your unconscious daydreams. When your monogamous partner lives separately, you start building routines that factor in that they are physically not there. So, for example, planning a meal doesn't include the "What do you feel like eating tonight?" question. No taste-testing will be shared.

On any day it's not unusual to drift in thought toward your sweetheart. When they're not there, that becomes an ache, a longing that you know will not be entirely satiated by a video chat—naked or otherwise.

Relationships are bound by both a mental and a physical connection. When the physical part is removed, what's left must be strong enough to carry the partnership forward. Being monogamous, and all its potential expansions, will reconfirm and reinforce the reasons why you were drawn to each other initially and why you chose to stay and build a life together.

Living apart together is a test for our relationship. Staying sexually, emotionally, and romantically monogamous are all separate agreements. Each LAT relationship is different, and each couple has different ideas of how things work. The foundation of our commitment to and trust in each other is what keeps it going, as well as the ability to give each other the freedom to grow and differentiate while staying connected.

These times are unprecedented. We are currently in a "she-cession," with over 5.4 million women having lost their jobs during the pandemic-induced recession (nearly one million more job losses than men).[21] While these numbers are bleak, they do indicate the need for change in the structure of our relationships. The need for a new type of expanded support for women and the need to outsource our childcare, our emotional support, and even our sexual partners has never been so clear.

Recently, Cambridge, Massachusetts, legalized polyamorous partnerships. They are the second city in the country to recognize polyamory as a domestic partnership between three or more people. They now define domestic partners as "the entity formed by two or more persons" who are not related. The only requirement is that the partners are "in a relationship of mutual support, caring and commitment and intend to remain in such a relationship," are "not in a domestic partnership with others outside this partnership," and "consider themselves to be a family."[22]

These people are monogamous within their partnership, with their partners, and consider themselves a family. And they do not have to live together. The language removes the requirement that all individuals in a domestic partnership must reside together.

The ordinance was created with the Polyamory Legal Advocacy Coalition, an association supported by the Chosen Family Law Center, the Harvard Law School LGBTQ+ Advocacy Clinic, and members of the American Psychological Association's Committee on Consensual Non-Monogamy, a group that advocates for legal recognition for polyamorous partnerships and other types of "non-nuclear families."

Alexander Chen of the Harvard Law School LGBTQ+ Advocacy Clinic said in a statement, "Non-nuclear families—such as single parents supported by relatives, step-families, open adoption families, multi-generational families, multi-parent families, and polyamorous families—have changed the landscape of American society, and yet, many of these diverse family structures are not protected or recognized by the law."[23]

Whatever the structure of your own relationship, it is most likely far from traditional, and is based instead on your personal needs. The common denominator, instead of traditional monogamy, should be honesty.

Open monogamy, LAT relationships, open relationships, and polyamory all depend on partners being open and honest. There's no hiding or cheating and the rules can be updated often. You should discuss your "open monogamy" agreement every time there is a change in your relationship.

We Do It for Love

Those who make the decision to marry, once, twice, or even a third time despite the ultimate commitment of marriage—instead of just living together—say love was the dominant factor in their decision to be legally married.[24]

Yet, only one-in-five adults in the United States say getting married leads to a fulfilling life, according to 2019 study. Marriage, in the traditional sense, is not vital for happiness.[25]

Perhaps it takes more than just committing to another person to be happily married. Maybe it takes a constant conversation, a reevaluation of what each individual wants, and a crossing of the bridge to meet the other. Marriage is not magic. Getting married doesn't solve problems and it's not a protection against infidelity. If you choose to enter a committed relationship, you are making a revolutionary step in your life. All the risks and difficulties, emotional heartache, and deep introspection that's required to be with another person take courage. It isn't easy to love another person and honor their needs as well as your own, to find the balance between what is right for you and what will work for them. Finding empathy and validating your partner while also noticing how you project your frustration onto them and being aware of your own shortcomings are all high-level skills.

Loving someone is not simple. It's never been easy. These days when we expect to live longer and stay sexual well into old age, it is more complicated than ever before. We want a primary partner, a love relationship, and we want the exciting energy of new relationships, new connections, and new sexual experiences. We want it all. Can it work? How do we work through our fears and our concerns? How do we make it happen without leaving any broken hearts in our wake?

Can Open Monogamy Work for Us?

Before you approach your partner with the possibility of changing your monogamy agreement, ask yourself:

Is our relationship solid enough to
withstand open monogamy?

Do we have old hurt or betrayal we need to
clear up before we open our monogamy?

Should we see a therapist to help
us open our relationship?

Do I want to welcome love relationships
with others into our marriage?

Do I want our relationship to come before all
others, or do I want it to be less hierarchical?

Am I aware of my own personal boundaries,
what I want or don't want?

Can I communicate with my partner and
share my personal boundaries with them?

Can I see myself dating and meeting
new people in this way?

If my partner told me they felt jealous,
would I change my behavior?

How would I feel if I were home alone
and my partner was out on a date?

Would I be honest with my partner and
share how I feel about their dating?

How will I handle being rejected or
ghosted by a potential new partner?

Would I be uncomfortable if my partner
gave someone more time or attention?

Could I ask my partner not to date
someone if I don't like them?

If they told me not to date someone,
could I give them *veto power*?

There are no wrong answers.

The most successful couples in open relationships are the ones who can
create a vision together, including a future of loving connection and communication. Couples who can create an agreement that is distinctive to
their personalized needs are the most satisfied with their arrangement and
seem to have the least amount of conflict. That means that things will
change as you grow. At times, your monogamy might be totally closed
and traditional, and at other times your relationship might include deeply
involved parallel relationships. One partner can be open, while the other
partner may be exclusive. All of these arrangements have one thing in
common: they are acceptable to both of you. You are the instigators of
your own revolution.

CHAPTER THREE

New Models of Monogamy

Anthropologist Wednesday Martin writes in her book *Untrue*, "There's now a pretty broad consensus that we evolved as cooperative breeders and, in our evolutionary history, we did not live in monogamous [pairings] . . . we lived in loose, rangy bands of people and we had multiple sex partners."

We have evolved to expect that marriage should be sexually monogamous with each partner desiring only one partner and living together till death. When in fact, this may not reflect the reality of monogamy today. Martin said, "Twenty percent of adults have practiced consensual non-monogamy at some point in their lives."

Back when the life expectancy was thirty-five years, we lived with a partner for an average of fourteen years. By the time we got bored, we were dead. Today, we live to be an average of seventy-eight years old, yet we are expected to live by the same old rules of marriage: get married, stay married, and stay monogamous.[2] We should be attracted to only that person and be desirous of only them, remaining true to them throughout our lifetime. Marriage, by this definition, is a lifetime of togetherness which could stretch to half a century or more.

There is no precedent for this model in history.

These days we live a longer, healthier life. We demand more from our intimate relationships. We want variety, excitement, eroticism, and adventure. Maybe because we have so many choices, we expect more from the person we "settle down" with. There are thousands of dating sites, over eight thousand worldwide and over 2,500 in the United States. We have access to an unlimited supply of potential partners at our fingertips every day. Therefore, choosing one permanent person can feel premature or restrictive and makes all the others feel dispensable.

DATING IN THE NEW MONOGAMY ERA

This paradox of choice is that it's hard to make a decision and stick to it without questioning if there is something better out there. The capacity to choose is always just a swipe away. When we are frustrated or angry with our current partner, it can feel like happiness with someone else is only a click away. With a never-ending variety of potential partners, in the end, we choose no one. It's like standing in the cereal aisle of a grocery store among dozens of different brands and bright attractive boxes. All of these options don't, in fact, make you buy more cereal. Studies show shoppers actually buy less, or none at all. The same thing can happen with dating and relationships. With all the alternatives available now, it is more difficult than ever to commit to just one partner.

As mate-seeking humans, we want stability, safety, attachment, and a contented life with a partner that we love. As a result, we find ourselves in a dilemma: we want to choose one mate and we want to shop around. We want long-term commitment but find it challenging to be with one person for what might be half or three quarters of a century or longer. How do we make a marriage work if we are expected to live long monogamous lives while there are so many alternative mating possibilities out there? Let's look at how real people are living some of the options available to us.

MODELS OF OPEN MONOGAMY

When you are ready to open your monogamy, you may be unsure of what you want to call it at first. You can call it anything you want. Don't try to label it if you don't want to. You don't have to put your relationship into a box and you don't have to give it a name. Just because other people have labels for their relationship doesn't mean you have to fit in to the current open relationship fashion. You don't have to be monogamish, consensually nonmonogamous, ethically nonmonogamous, open, swingers, or polyamorous. You don't have to be totally traditionally monogamous either. You can call yourselves and your agreement anything you want to. Be open to the possibilities and know that *you can change your minds anytime* and call it something else.

Let's look at some of the models or types of open monogamy. They may give you some idea of how to structure your own agreement.

Equality Model

In an open relationship the need for equality is crucial. The open monogamy model is based on being a couple—any kind of couple: gay, straight, bisexual, asexual, or pansexual—who consider themselves to be primary partners to each other. Their relationship is central even, when, and if they open it to others.

Between the primary partners there is no one partner that is more important; they are equal in power and share in the distribution of resources. They rely on each other for emotional and financial support which makes the risk of manipulation or coercion less. Both partners share in household decisions and decisions around parenting, although one may have more childcare responsibilities or take on more around the house. They both share responsibility for making their sex life successful, although one may want sex less or more often than the other. In open monogamy, the relationship between the partners is predominantly equal.

Some polyamorous couples describe the *equality model* as one where all partners have equal priority in the relationship, including outside partners. They share feelings, sex, and even household responsibilities equally.

Are Outside Relationships Equal?

The reality of being an outside partner to an open monogamy couple is that the primary couple is always central to one another. For someone on the outside coming in, this commitment can be confusing and sometimes hurtful. In some open relationships, there is an assumption that being brought into a couples' relationship ensures equal treatment. In many cases, the new partner may appear to have all of the same emotional, sexual, and companionate benefits and consideration that the primary partners have, and be made to feel just as important, but they will not have the status of a primary partner. Their connection should not be dismissed or minimized, but they may never have equal status in the relationship.

The longer the main couple has been together and the more commitment they've made to their marriage or partnership, the more likely that it will include some kind of legal contract, a mortgage, in-laws, children, and a whole history that came before the relationship was opened. In most cases, the relationship with an outside partner will not be equal but that doesn't mean it can't be special or unique.

In an open monogamy relationship, the couple works to keep their relationship central. Outside relationships are naturally secondary. This does not mean that outside relationships can't work or aren't important.

Couples interested in being polyamorous need to talk about a myriad of things, particularly when they first decide to try poly. You need to choose how to structure the relationship and discuss things like the roles additional partners will play. Are you looking for a second emotional partner, or do you want something sexual? Are you allowed to stay over at your second partner's house, or is that off-limits? How much time should you be spending with your second partner?

Discussing these difficult questions will ensure you and your partner are on the same page and can keep your existing relationship healthy while you explore new kinds of intimacy with other partners.

In a true equality model, all partners in the open relationship are equal. They have equal rights in the emotional relationship, equal status as sexual partners, and equal responsibility as co-parents. This model of open relationship is adapted in polyamorous relationships, where couples welcome in other romantic partners and may share the home and domestic responsibilities.

Romantic Monogamy

You may be monogamous romantically and open sexually. This means that your emotional connection remains true to your partner, but you have an agreement that you can be sexual with other people. That might mean you are sexual with other people alongside your partner or separately. But in *romantic monogamy*, neither of you will fall in love with someone else or let yourself have romantic feelings outside of your marriage. This would mean that you are committed to letting each other know if that were to begin to happen and/or stopping yourself before you got to that place of emotional connection with any outside partner.

Sexual Monogamy

Sexual monogamy means you agree that sex only happens between the two of you. First, you have to define what sex means. Is it touching, kissing, being naked, touching to orgasm, or oral sex? Be clear with each other about what you mean by sexual monogamy. If you are going to commit to being monogamous sexually and not sleep with anyone else, have intercourse, or touch another person, does that mean you will do sexual things together in front of people, or watch other people have sex, but only when you are together? Do you have a rule where these things have to happen if together, or can some of these things happen when you are alone or traveling? And if something happens, will you tell each other?

The Difference Between Romantic Monogamy and Sexual Monogamy

The difference between romantic and sexual monogamy might seem slight or dramatically different. Think about what it would look like to you. Would you have nights when you could be with other people, lovers' nights, or outside partner nights, or will you keep separate rooms so you can have the privacy to do what you want with whomever you want?

Is touching a romantic gesture or a sexual gesture? What is the line between touching a friend and touching for flirting or making a sexual overture? How do you talk about your concerns if one thing crosses over to another? The communication tools in this book will help you ask questions like:

What kind of touch am I okay with outside of our relationship?

What if I am uncomfortable with you
touching someone else sexually?

Do I want romantic or sexual monogamy?

What would it be like to have a night apart
from each other with other people?

What is the difference between privacy and secrecy?

POLYAMORY, PRIMARIES, AND SECONDARIES

Leif met with me by Zoom to talk about his open monogamy relationship.

He volunteered to tell me about his history and his partner and their experience with communication and family.

When Leif met Eugenia, he had been married twice and widowed for several years. He considers himself polyamorous and "definitely has one primary partner."

His primary partner, Eugenia, is "not 100 percent sure she's poly," but she mostly is. She has been negotiating this relationship and wrapping her mind around it from the beginning. "I told her on the second or third date that I wasn't going to be monogamous."

Leif has a young son and no interest in getting married again. He did, however, want a committed relationship. He likes being with someone he loves and has no problem being with a primary partner. He prefers it. When he started dating Eugenia, he was very clear that monogamy, in the traditional sense, was not going to work for him.

Eugenia was unsure how she felt about polyamory. With a childhood history of emotional abandonment she was uncertain, but she liked Leif a lot. They sought a poly-compatible therapist (a couple's therapist who has experience working with polyamory and open relationships) and talked about some of the challenges, possibilities, potential problems, and benefits that Leif was proposing.

Seven years later, they are still together and happy. Both have *secondary partners*. The primary and secondary structure is essential for Eugenia's security, according to Leif. When she feels insecure, it's because she doesn't feel primary. Her triggers are abandonment and insecurity. Leif bragged about her, adding, "She has a great capacity to work through her feelings. She is insightful and brave to be doing this."

"Is there a way it could be better?" I asked.

"I just wish she could relax into it. Have sex with others when she wants without worrying about me. Choose not to have sex with others without worrying about me. Know that when I have sex with others, it is not because I am unhappy with her, nor is she, or our relationship, deficient."

I asked, "How do you handle your monogamy to both partners or all of your partners?"

"We are both monogamous to both primary and secondary partners. I don't cheat," he said. "Secondaries have rights too. I have had some long-lasting and significant secondary relationships."

They want to know each other's *metamours* and want everyone in their families to get along. It doesn't always work out that way.

Metamour

The meaning of a metamour in polyamory circles is the lover of one's partner. A metamour is not someone with whom you have a direct sexual or romantic relationship; they are your partner's partner. In kitchen table poly, you may spend a lot of time with this person. They may spend the night at your house with your partner. They may become part of your extended, intentional family.

Kitchen Table Poly

Kitchen table poly refers to people in primary and secondary relationships that feel comfortable hanging out together. They are able to be together in the same house, sitting around the kitchen table having tea, for instance, or a meal. For those who prefer kitchen table poly, being friends is essential.

One of the challenges of Leif and Eugenia's relationship is that Eugenia's current partner doesn't want to meet Leif. He would like them all to be part of the same pod, including Eugenia's partner. He would like them all to practice *kitchen table poly*.

Leif said, "With my ex-wife, she knew about my other partners. We were open about them."

Leif and Eugenia have a version of kitchen table poly, because she knows his partners, and is okay with them being at his house, but Leif said, "I'd like it if she would get along better with my play partners."

What makes it work, he said, is that "Eugenia is very good at talking about her feelings. Nothing festers."

Talking about everything is an integral part of their relationship. Leif and Eugenia talk about their agreement and make changes as needed. Some things are easier than others. The negotiation has grown more comfortable over time.

There is less tension in their relationship than there used to be. Leif said, "I'm better at talking and processing than I used to be."

I asked him what he wished he had done differently in the relationship. Leif said, "In the beginning, I had more outside partners. I wasn't good at setting that up skillfully; I might have been sabotaging it. I'm still learning—I haven't always been good at it."

At the beginning of his relationship with Eugenia, Leif met his secondary partner, Laura. Eugenia had been divorced for a long time and had some experience with open relationships but hadn't tried polyam.

"Her kids were grown, and she seemed ready to experiment. I introduced her to the word poly, and she worked through some of her assumptions about what that meant," Leif said.

After months of sheltering in place in separate houses, Eugenia is moving in with Leif. They have always had independent households and have never tried living together, nor have they had outside partners living with them. Their relationship seems to be moving to a new level.

Leif isn't into quick, overnight relationships. He had one outside partner prior to Laura, which lasted for twenty-two years, longer than his two marriages.

"A weekend together is perfect," he said. "It's one of the things I like about poly, it gives you a way to enjoy the good parts of someone or a relationship."

Being in an open monogamy relationship doesn't mean you have commitment or intimacy issues. Leif is open to being with someone for the long haul and Eugenia is not shy about her capacity for connection. Being poly, for both of them, is about love and family.

I asked if he and Eugenia had a flexible agreement about how many partners they could have in their relationship. He said they had long ago moved from "coercive agreements" to flexibility.

"We check things out with each other. We have never really had to negotiate. We are not into swinging or casual sex, so we don't put each other at risk. I've met some people, and they've been serious relationships, some not as much. The best part is there is more love with more people and more excitement. The worst part is there are more breakups and more drama, lots of drama.

"Falling in love is lovely and breaking up sucks—just like in mono relationships. I'd like to think I've gotten better at the breaking up. I've been poly since I was fourteen. I'm proud of the fact that I'm friends with all the people I used to sleep with, I'm even still friends with Eugenia's ex.

"If you love someone enough to make it a capital "R" relationship, it doesn't mean that you can't be friends. Just because you couldn't make it work doesn't mean they aren't a good person. For instance, one of my ex-lovers wanted to be first, she wanted to be primary and didn't want to be secondary. That wasn't going to work for me. But we are still good friends."

I asked him to define a small "r" relationship. He said, "A small 'r' relationship is a buddy for sex only. Lately, I have more play partners but that's not a matter of preference exactly, more like an opportunity, and lack of drive to find another big relationship.

"I believe in taking each person and each potential relationship as they are. I don't think it's productive to go out hunting for a preconceived thing. Some poly newbies make this mistake; the classic is the *unicorn hunter*. When I meet somebody I'm interested in, I am okay with not knowing what might happen. Maybe we'll be friends, and that's good. Maybe we'll do sex play, and maybe it will become a relationship, perhaps not. I'm okay with taking it as it goes to see what happens.

"One of my closest friends, and now one of my partner's good friends too, is a woman I've propositioned a few times over the years. She said no, and that's fine. Another of my closest friends is an ex-lover. Being friends doesn't mean it is a failed relationship. These are all relationships that have found the right level."

Unicorn

A *unicorn* is a single bisexual who is available for sex with a couple but is not interested in an emotional commitment, and therefore not seen as a threat to the marriage. A unicorn is usually a female. Some couples go unicorn hunting online to search for this illusive female.

Polycule

The word *polycule* refers to everyone in a sexual, emotional, or romantic relationship network or structure. A polycule is connected intimately but may not be kitchen table poly or fluid bonded. There are many variations on this, and it can be called different things, including: pod, family, community, constellation, network, tribe, *triad*, quad, or *thruple* (see glossary).

Today, at sixty years old, Leif loves Eugenia and still considers her his primary partner. "We still love each other even when we are fed up."

His advice for people who want to try an open monogamy relationship? "Relax. Ride the escalator to the next phase, and don't worry too much."

IS IT SAFE TO OPEN MY RELATIONSHIP?

In a recent study published in the *Social Psychology and Personality Science* journal, researchers found that opening up a relationship had no negative impact on life satisfaction or relationship quality in romantic partnerships. The study shows that open relationships can be a healthy, viable option for some couples.

In this study of 233 people, they compared the relational, sexual, and personal well-being of couples before and after they opened up their monogamy to couples who remained monogamous throughout the study. Not only did they find that there were no differences in well-being before and after people opened up their relationship, but the couples who opened their relationships had a significant increase in sexual satisfaction. The study showed that opening a relationship can create new erotic energy within the marriage.[3]

For many couples, open monogamy is a practical option. For others, it can be unappealing to try to stretch the boundaries of their current agreement. All consensual agreements between consenting adults should be normalized.

Our next couple, Gail and Gene, are models of a long-term, committed, open monogamy relationship.

GAIL AND GENE

Gail and Gene volunteered to be interviewed for this book. They are in their late fifties and have been married for thirty-six years. They live in Colorado in a rambling three-story carriage house on a small horse farm surrounded by trees and a swimming pool. Gail and Gene are both artists and work from home in a shared outdoor studio that was built onto the back of their house. Gail identifies as bisexual, with Gene claiming to be "slightly gender fluid." They have raised three children, all of whom have grown and left the house.

Gail and Gene are in an open monogamy relationship. They consider each other as primary and see their marriage as their priority. "We prioritize each other's needs," Gail told me in our interview in her kitchen.

"Our relationship is crucial, and we prioritize our family above any of our outside needs. Family will always come first," she said.

Gene and Gail defer to each other when discussing what is comfortable and what is not. When I asked them to describe their open monogamy relationship, Gail said, "Go ahead, Gene, you answer the question."

Gene said, "It's true, our relationship always comes first. We check in with each other. It is not *relationship anarchy*."

Relationship Anarchy

Some couples approach their consensual nonmonogamy with a relationship anarchy structure, or a nonhierarchical, political perspective. It is strictly anti-monogamous, with a strong affiliation toward a lack of relational labels. The relationship anarchists don't want to call their partners primary or secondary or inside or outside, and they insist that relationship models repress the individual, are coercive, and are based on ownership while oppressing freedom. They value equality above all.

Gail said, "I have other partners that are important, but this is a hierarchical relationship. Gene is the most important person to me. He will always come first. We check in with each other about going out with other people, or if we want to go out on dates, we always talk about it first, before we let anything happen."

I asked Gene if they had the power of vetoing potential partners. "We trust each other's judgment," he said. "While we each hold veto power over who the other may date, we take great care in how we look at this issue. Our *redline* is if we are going to be with other people, those people have to be honest and open with their partners. There has to be no dishonesty. We can't be with outside partners that are cheating. We aren't cheating, and we can't be with cheaters."

Gail and Gene's open monogamy relationship started ten years ago. Gene met a woman at a gallery in Miami and she and Gene started a three-week affair. It was an emotional affair, and he became attached to this woman who he found exotic and exciting. They talked every day on the phone, texting and growing close. Things had not been sexual, yet, but feelings were heating up. He realized he couldn't hide things from Gail and didn't want to lie to her. He decided to tell her, but only after she asked him if something was going on.

Gail said, "He seemed distant and strange. I asked him what was wrong. He told me he had met a woman. He loved her. I was pissed."

"I felt really bad about hurting Gail," Gene said. "But I liked my relationship with this woman, let's call her Dawn. I appreciated her attention, she made me feel young and attractive and it was great to be with her. She understood my painting, and we talked for hours. But I felt awful that I had been keeping this from Gail. Nothing like this had ever happened to us before."

Gail said, "Gene and I had a lot of conversations about it. We went to therapy. I was hurt. I didn't like that he had lied to me, kept things a secret. It took a while, but eventually I understood. He had needed something that I couldn't give him. It was the newness, the excitement, it was something bright and shiny. No matter what I did or said, I was never going to be that for him."

"It wasn't because I didn't love Gail anymore—quite the contrary," Gene said. "In fact, during this time we were having more sex than we ever had."

Gail said, "Yes, and better sex too. The best." They smiled at each other. She continued, "In therapy we talked a lot. We talked about opening our relationship. We wondered what it would be like. We decided we each needed permission to just explore a little."

I asked Gail if she wanted Gene to stop seeing Dawn or if she gave him the green light to keep up that relationship. Did she feel she had no other choice? I wanted to know if she felt coerced into an open relationship because Gene was pushing to continue his affair, but now with permission.

She said, "It was okay with me if he wanted to go ahead and sleep with her. I came to terms with that. I knew no matter what, he wouldn't leave me. It wasn't the sex with her that bothered me. It was all the texting and the amount of time he spent on their relationship. He was always thinking about her and talking to her so frequently. That was the betrayal."

Gene said, "I understood that. Time is Gail's language of love. Back then, I was definitely obsessing over Dawn, and we texted constantly." Gene nodded and Gail shot him a look, and then rolled her eyes.

"Yeah, you were obsessing, a little," she laughed. "I felt left out."

Gail said, "I had to be honest with myself, too. I understood Gene's attraction to her. Dawn was different than me; she was small, dark, and foreign. I knew he was attracted to that difference; that was never going to be me."

Gene said, "Plus, I didn't have a lot of sexual experiences prior to our marriage. I was new at all of it. I felt like I was making up for lost time."

I asked how they came to their agreement. Gail said, "We talked about what it would be like. I got over my feelings about Dawn.

And we gave each other permission to be with other people. It turned out that it was a good thing to do. It was kind of a sexual turn-on to do that."

Gene agreed. "Totally."

She looked at him and said softly, "It made me love you more."

I asked Gail how opening their marriage worked for her. Did she want to see other people at that point?

She said, "At first Gene and I were having too much sex for me to think about actually seeing other people. Just by talking about opening up we were having more sex than ever before, like twice a day. I think I was trying to exhaust him." She laughed and he agreed.

"It's true," he said.

I said it sounds like *mate guarding*. Mate guarding is when you try to have so much sex with your partner that they are too tired to be with anyone outside of the marriage. It is a way of keeping away competition. Mate guarding is a common defense in the animal kingdom when a mate feels threatened by outside competitors.[4]

She laughed and said, "It was really the first time in our relationship where we had such great sex."

I looked at Gene to see what he thought. "We finally had an empty nest, too. It was probably the first time we had been alone in twenty years. So, yeah, it was good. Really good," he said.

I asked what finally ended Gene's relationship with Dawn.

"It was Dawn's inability to be honest," he said.

Now that everything was out in the open with Gail, Gene found it disingenuous to lie about anything. He told Dawn the truth, that Gail was fine with them seeing each other as long as he was open about everything. Dawn, to his surprise, was not happy about this arrangement. She wanted Gene to lie to Gail, to keep secrets.

I wondered aloud if keeping their affair a secret was the only way Dawn could be intimate with Gene. "Maybe," he said. "She liked that we were sneaking around. I did not."

I said, "Maybe Dawn was looking for tension to make things exciting. Some people seek illicitness, and the transparency of an honest, open monogamy makes them uncomfortable. Dawn may not have wanted to just be an accessory to your marriage, either. Perhaps she was hoping for something more, that maybe you would leave your marriage and be with her; maybe she didn't like being secondary."

Gene said, "I really liked her a lot. But I wasn't going to leave Gail to be with Dawn."

Shortly after Gene broke up with Dawn, Gail met a woman she was interested in both sexually and romantically. With Gene's approval, Gail began her outside relationship, a romantic and sexual relationship that would last for over four years.

Gene said, "I was okay with it. I trust our relationship. I know we aren't going to leave each other."

Gene said for many couples, trusting the relationship is what makes open monogamy work. He said he trusts their relationship. Couples who rely on their relationship and their agreement know that this is what makes their foundation strong. It is less likely that they will break up over monogamy betrayals or misunderstandings. They don't have to rely on trusting each other because they know that people are fallible and make mistakes. They rely on their relationship and their ability to communicate and create an agreement that can be changed to fit their constantly evolving lives. By relying on the agreement, they have something concrete to return to, and in making this their priority, they find more leeway to explore outside of it.

Gene has slowed down his experimentation, while Gail finds she has been exploring more often. Gene said, "If I am going to explore other partners, I want love. I am tired of searching, always looking. I'm tired of dating."

"What's it like, looking for partners?" I asked.

"I used to be on OkCupid," he said. "I would tell people shortly after meeting them that I was in an open relationship. Sometimes they were fine with it, sometimes not. I rarely connected deeply with anyone. So, I'd have to start again. It takes so much time. I don't like the time it took."

I asked if he had tried any other websites, places for married people to find dates, for instance. He said, "I don't like sites like

Ashley Madison because their whole thing is based on dishonesty. My foundation, my values, are all about honesty. The whole foundation of my life is honesty, family, and my marriage with Gail. Why would I want to be in a relationship with someone who I know for a fact is lying?"

Gene is now on FetLife, a website for people exploring *kink* and *BDSM* relationships, a type of play that might involve bondage, discipline, sadomasochism, submission, and/or dominance. "I am exploring a little more kink. Maybe I will meet someone on that site. I'm not in any hurry."

I asked them, "What is the biggest challenge of your open monogamy relationship?"

Gene said, "I get tired of the competition."

I asked, "Tired of the competition with other men?"

"No, this competition I feel with Gail, the competition to find similar sexual experiences and always having a new partner. I don't have the energy she does. She can have several sexual partners in a week. I want to really get to know someone, have a real relationship. Gail's the exact opposite. She doesn't really want to get emotionally involved."

"Yeah, I just want to have a fun time," she said. "But I am pretty discerning. I don't have sex at parties or gatherings or anything. I am kind of a private person."

Gene said, "The hardest part for both of us, I think, is that after Gail gets home from a date, I want to talk about it, and she doesn't."

She said, "He has feelings about me dating other people, but he just says, 'Yes, go ahead.' He has feelings about the 'yes,' but he won't tell me what they are. So, I go out and have fun. I wish he would talk to me more about his feelings."

"Okay," he said. "I'll tell you how I feel right now. You have too many people you're involved with."

"Oh, well, thank you for telling me that, at least that's honest," she said.

Gene looked at me. "I'm fine, actually. Open monogamy works for us. I'm just glad she's not really attached to any of them."

I asked them both how they handle jealousy. Gail said, "You just suck up the jealousy. It's not magic. Just suck it up."

Gene said, "I'm jealous of that energy that she's not sharing. Sometimes. She doesn't bring home the energy. I'm not jealous of the sex."

The best part for Gail? "I'm getting the sexual experiences I want. The sex life between us has improved and grown to this new place. I am *squirting* now," she tells me and laughs.

Gene said, "We have evolved and managed our relationship, together."

Gail said, "We set a higher bar for our sex. We are even doing some *flogging*. It feels more integrated."

When I asked them about their vision for the future of their monogamy, Gail said, "I don't see myself ever being monogamous again."

IS MONOGAMY NATURAL?

Some people claim that they are "just not born to be monogamous." This would somehow imply that biologically we as a species aren't inclined to choose a mate and be faithful throughout a lifetime. Or, that certain humans are oriented toward monogamy and others aren't.

"Are we meant to be monogamous?" is not a simple question. To look at whether or not we are "born" monogamous we have to examine human fertility and sexual behavior as they relate to the way we form family bonds. We are not "born" knowing how to eat with a fork, yet as humans, we can learn. We learn and process and grow and adapt in relation to our bonds with others. We are able to form all types of behavioral strategies to get by in the world and to connect. We eat in a manner that is socially agreed upon, and we mate in a way that protects our partners and our young.

But we have choices. We can choose how we eat, and we can choose how we mate. With the studies in behavioral genetics, molecular genetics, neuroendocrinology, and cross-species analysis we can look at monogamy as an evolutionary adaptation. We choose to be monogamous. Or we choose not to be.

Scientists, anthropologists, and researchers have a lot to say about the neural basis for pair bonding and monogamy as it relates to biology and human behavior.

Larry J. Young, who works in behavioral neuroscience and psychiatric disorders, said that only 5 percent of mammals are monogamous.[5] He defines monogamy not as lifelong exclusivity with a single mate, however; he said monogamy is selective (not exclusive) mating, which means "a shared nesting area, and biparental care." Monogamy is selecting a mate to make a home with and have children, but not necessarily to be exclusively sexual with.

Over ninety bird species form pair bonds and raise offspring together, but they only stick to that plan for one season at a time. The next season they select a new partner. For those species assumed to be monogamous (geese, for example), DNA sampling of their eggs has proven that extra-pair copulation does happen. Even geese, the birds we have long assumed to be monogamous, don't exactly mate exclusively. The female will search out extra males to mate with while he is out searching for food. But she only shares her nest with her partner.

In the mammal kingdom, the female is only sexually receptive during ovulation. But humans are different than all other animals. We have sex not just for reproduction, but for pleasure and for connection. In humans, sex can happen throughout the female cycle, not just when a woman is fertile. This capacity for sexual activity throughout the female cycle "stimulates the neural circuits responsible for maintaining the pair bond, preserving the strength of the bond over time," according to scientists.[6]

This could mean that we like to have sex to connect, to attach, and for pleasure. It doesn't have much to do with whether we are or are not born monogamous. It means we are born with the potential for multiple sexual partners, yes. And we are born to seek sexual pleasure. Whether we find that in back-to-back seasons with different mates, with multiple partners at one time, or with one partner for life is likely determined by how we connect.

SOLO POLY

Some people who identify as polyamorous prefer to live independently and don't want to commit to a primary partner. That does not mean they don't want relationships. A 2016 study found that 20 percent of single people have participated in a consensually nonmonogamous relationship.[7]

Solo poly is a term used to describe a person who is committed to being single but identifies with a polyamorous orientation. They may describe themselves as single, autonomous, and unwilling to commit to one person but available to date other poly people or pods of people. They may not want to be in a primary partnership, but are open to many romantic and sexual partners. There is controversy over the term solo poly, as some find this description a cover for anyone who can't commit or isn't interested in attaching. That may or may not be true. Solo poly is a self-ascribed orientation that describes an individual who identifies as poly in their orientation and is not interested in a traditional monogamous relationship. They value their freedom and tend to lean toward relationship anarchy.

Relationship anarchists agree to stay together with someone for as long as it is working for them. They don't make promises to stay together forever and live in the moment, preferring to work with their current emotional status. The anarchists reject any external socially imposed obligations or rules for their relationships.

This means that their connections are based on love, respect, and choice. They stay with someone out of a desire to be together, and as long as they are happy, it works. If it becomes unstable, they put in the time to communicate and try to work it out, as a lot of people do in open or consensually nonmonogamous relationships. Just like open monogamy, in solo poly, all obligations to partners are open to change and are fluid and flexible with time and circumstance.

Solo poly status can be conflated with relationship anarchy. Solo polys are the folks that were called the "lifetime confirmed bachelor or bachelorette" in the past or might be seen as having "attachment" or "commitment issues" by those who are not familiar with their orientation. Solo polys can have many meaningful relationships that serve them well but may avoid interdependency.

Sociological researcher Elisabeth "Eli" Sheff said, "Some solo polys say that they are their own primaries, either because they find autonomy compelling or they are repelled by the primary-partnership relationship model."[8]

Being single and poly can mean that you see yourself (or others see you) as a "unicorn." A solo poly can welcome this type of relationship or resent it. If a solo poly person prefers an unattached purely sexual lifestyle, they may be open to multiple sexual experiences with multiple partners without emotional attachment, which we would commonly call "swinging," if the person was in a relationship and not solo.

Over three-quarters of people who identify as swingers say their life is "exciting." Swingers are seen as more adventurous and more open to new experiences.[9] Some single people who identify as solo poly may think of themselves as a swinger, or as someone who prefers multiple partners, not just for sex but for romantic and emotional connections.

LAMIKA

I interviewed Lamika, a retired, sixty-eight-year-old biracial Hawaiian woman living on Kauai. She is not solo poly as such, because she identifies as being in a primary relationship with her boyfriend Kai, but she is currently in an open monogamy relationship, identifies as bisexual, and lives alone. Lamika is widowed and has no children of her own but calls Kai's son her stepson.

She defines her current relationship with Kai as primary and hierarchical. They are primary partners and while he has outside partners, she doesn't have anyone she's seeing right now.

"I was not poly when we met," she told me. "I really knew very little about it at the time. I sort of knew from another guy I had dated that poly meant 'I'm not exclusive, I date and sleep with other people.' But I had been monogamous most of my life. I had one nine-year relationship where we divorced and my second husband of twenty-two years died."

I asked her, "Did you know right away that you wanted to be in some kind of open relationship with Kai or were you expecting something more traditional?"

She said, "Kai had been poly all of his life, with multiple relationships before, during, and after his previous marriage. He explained that he wanted our relationship to come first, but I was having a hard time with it. I had never done this before."

"It sounds like it was all new to you when you met him," I said.

Lamika said, "Yes, and it was hard. It took great effort to be with him. He said he was looking for a primary partner but it was confusing. When I met him, he was with two other women, one he had been with for over twenty years and one for about two years. I was concerned. I asked him, 'Am I tertiary?' I didn't know what I was to him. He wanted me to meet his other women. I told him, 'I'll meet your family,' but I didn't want to meet his girlfriends. It was so complicated. I was totally oblivious to what poly was going to be like. There were a lot of dos and don'ts right off the bat. It was very intense."

"What made you stick it out?" I asked.

"We fell in love. Well, that caused problems with his other relationships. But we read a lot of books together. We would highlight things in the book. We read *The Ethical Slut* and *Opening Up*. We went to poly conventions and we talked a lot. At one point I went into therapy to deal with all of my poly 'issues.'"

I asked, "What do you mean, poly issues? Was the relationship structure not working for you?"

Lamika said, "For years I felt like I wasn't doing poly 'right.' I had too many questions and I wanted too many things, but I didn't say what I wanted, I didn't stand up for myself. Finally, I grew more confident. I have needs. I started to stand up for what was important to me. It was a rollercoaster for a while, but eventually we went to couples therapy together and that was really good. It worked for a while. And then COVID came. We stopped seeing other people. We sheltered in place in our own homes, two different homes. I feel committed to him, being there for him. I don't know if his other partners would be there for him like I am. I am not sure he appreciates that. I am there for him, I really support him emotionally."

"Do you ever date anyone else or have any other partners, or is it just Kai?" I asked.

She said, "It was two years into our relationship before I started seeing anyone else. I had reconnected with an old boyfriend but we haven't seen each other since COVID. I saw this guy for two years, kind of a friend with benefits. Then, he met someone else and said he wanted to be exclusive with her but wanted to still get together with me occasionally. I would rather be with someone where all the cards are on the table, where there is integrity. I've met men in the past that said, 'I'm open, but I don't tell my wife.' I don't go further with them. If they say things like 'I do this because my wife doesn't have sex with me,' I don't buy it."

I said, "It sounds like you really value integrity."

"I have a lot of integrity, and that's what you want when you do this. In my thirties I was very promiscuous; now I care about who I sleep with. I want there to be a heart connection. I want to care about someone and feel safe with them and have them care about me if I'm going to have sex with them."

"Is Kai still seeing other people?" I asked.

"He is still seeing one other woman. The three of us have played together, but nothing lately. We talked about her coming over when I'm not there. I don't feel threatened by her, but I don't really want to be there. For now we are keeping things just between us. She might come over again after six weeks or so."

"What's the most challenging part of this relationship?" I asked.

"The hardest part of this is Kai's moodiness. I am a helper, an empath. I have to work to not lose myself in this relationship. I'm there for him during challenging times. To be honest, I'm not sure he would be there for me. When his wife had cancer years ago, he actually still had other lovers. I don't think that would work for me. Another thing that is really hard is the lack of consistency. We will make plans, for instance, and he backs off. That part's hard."

Lamika continued, "I've also been there when Kai flipped for someone else. All that new relationship energy. When that happened, he forgot all of our agreements. That really didn't work for me. That's when we started therapy. We have grown since then, but those wounds are still there. There are scars and I still have fears. That to me is the hardest part."

I asked, "What are your redlines in this relationship now?"

"My redlines are we both always have to have safe sex with others. And we have to tell each other about having sex with other people. We have to be honest. We don't have a veto policy; neither of us wants that."

"Have you ever had reason to request that Kai stop seeing someone?" I asked.

"There was a time when he was seeing a woman in the company where I work. I was scared that she would break my confidentiality. I told him, 'You cannot share anything with this person, not about me.' He finally stopped seeing her. It was pretty uncomfortable. I didn't feel safe. I didn't trust her; she had a reputation of causing problems in the organization. I was worried about confidentiality. But he ended it willingly."

"What works for you about this open monogamy?" I asked.

"What works for us? I like that we talk, we talk deeply. With my husband I thought we had a good sex life and talked about sex, but not compared to Kai and I. We are really close, we talk about things a lot. I think that's really healthy; we both feel it's the healthiest relationship we've ever had. It's the most we've ever been able to communicate. It's not easy communication, but it's good communication."

"Who knows about your open relationship?" I asked.

Lamika said, "My family's definitely not open to the idea. My father might have gone out on my mother, but no one ever talked about it. I told my sister, she's the conservative one. She said 'do not' tell our other sister. I wasn't surprised. It's not something I can talk about with my family. I have told some close friends of mine."

"Does Kai's family know?"

"His whole family is poly, his sister and his brother. In fact, he thinks his parents were in an open relationship but never said. In his family, being poly is the answer to everything. Or, at least it's the answer to a lot of situations. If you're frustrated with your partner or you're horny, just go have sex with other people. That's not how I would do it."

"Are you a more private person?" I asked.

"Keeping my privacy makes me feel protected. I also just don't want the hassle. I was a teacher for thirty-eight years. No one knew. It's tricky to manage privacy, but it's easier in the long run."

"What advice do you have for other couples, especially if something doesn't work or if something goes wrong?"

She said, "Really figure out what you specifically want and communicate that. See if that is compatible before you try anything. And if you are a man, don't assume that if a woman is poly it automatically means she wants to sleep with you. Lots of the men I meet think that's the case. It's not true. I'm not going to sleep with you."

"I know this is a stressful time for you, with COVID."

She said, "Since COVID I feel like we should all just go for it, just go all the way in our relationships. My ex died of prostate cancer. You just never know how long you have with someone."

CHAPTER FOUR

How Do We Start?

Our capacity for connection is not just about having sex. Humans can maintain pair bonds beyond one season and beyond biparental care, after the kids grow up and leave the nest. We attach to a shared nesting area and most of the time, loathe to give it up. But, in order to make a relationship work for many, many seasons in the same nest with the same person, we have to learn to connect and create good relationship skills. If we don't want to mate exclusively, but we want to stay with the same mate, we have to balance extra-pair copulations with our innate human potential for really messing things up. To avoid this potential for messing up our primary relationships, we need special skill sets. We have to learn higher-human skills; we have to have insight, we have to see our own blind spots, and we have to be able to articulate our emotions and empathize with our partner.

CELINE AND PENA

Celine and Pena were in therapy to talk about opening their marriage. They had some issues that had to be worked out before they could continue that conversation and wanted to know how to work through some of their basic relationship conflicts. They came to therapy to practice empathy and validation. Without these skills, opening their marriage would only cause more problems between them.

Celine and Pena argued most days. Celine had a full-time job working in a hospital, and in the evenings she came home and made dinner and took care of their two kids. Pena was a writer and spent all day and most evenings closed off in his study on his laptop. Celine felt lonely, overwhelmed, and overburdened. Pena felt stressed about money and anxious that he wouldn't meet his manuscript deadline. When Pena and Celine came to therapy, Celine said,

"We love each other, but we are in constant conflict and I want a new kind of relationship."

Pena agreed. "Things are stressful at home."

Celine said, "I wonder if an open relationship might be the answer?"

Pena said, "I don't know how that will help. Won't we just fight more?"

Celine looked at him, her eyes tired. She still wore her scrubs from work and her face mask hung heavy around her throat. She said, "I want a more equal relationship. I want Pena to help around the house and with the kids and I want to go out more with my friends. Maybe it means dating other people, I don't know. But right now, I can't take it anymore. My stress level is through the roof. I feel alone in this relationship." She started to cry.

Pena's face grew red, he balled up his fists, and his jaw grew tight. "I am working hard too," he said, his voice gruff, bouncing off the walls of my small office. "You are not understanding what I go through, you don't get me at all . . ."

"I know you don't want to argue," I said. "Let's work on empathizing with each other's feelings. Neither of you are wrong here; it sounds like you are really longing to be heard and understood."

"She doesn't understand me," Pena said.

"He doesn't care how hard I work," Celine said. "I want an open marriage. I am done."

"An open marriage is not the same as a separation," I said. "Before you can discuss opening your relationship or changing anything, it's important to feel heard. First, let's try this:

Each of you can try to empathize with what the other is going through. You don't have to agree or forgive or explain or apologize. Just try to understand and validate the other person's experience, so they will know you really see them and are aware of what it's like to be in their shoes. Can we try?"

They both nodded.

"Start with the words 'I understand that ____' or 'It makes sense that ____' and see if you can let the other person know that you know how they feel, not just how you feel."

Celine began, "I get that you are working hard. I know you are in the middle of your book and things are difficult for you right now. I do understand. It makes sense that you have to hide away right now. I know you get stressed when you are writing, but I feel like you don't understand what I am going through."

"Did she get your feelings, Pena?"

"I guess, sort of."

"Okay, let's see if you can empathize with her."

Pena said, "I get that you are working in that hospital all day and it is a scary, crazy environment. You are risking your life every day and then you come home and you just want to relax. It's hard with the kids, and we don't have any help." He looked at her closely. "You must be so tired. I am so sorry."

Celine began to cry. "I am not that tired, Pena. I am lonely. If you can't pay attention to me, I thought maybe I could meet someone else, someone who can share their love with me. You don't have time for me."

I said, "An open relationship is not a way to fix something that is broken at home. If you are going to try a more flexible monogamy, you first have to be able to talk about the things that bother you and the things you want—all of it, with empathy. Before you try to open your marriage, you will have to practice this kind of talking, learning how to empathize and understand each other's feelings and how to deal with your conflicts. Otherwise, you won't be able to resolve the issues that come up in your marriage. And an open marriage is even more complicated."

If you are feeling overwhelmed by the prospect of this much change in your relationship, come back to the basics. Open monogamy works the same way as any relationship, through good communication, creating mutual respect, setting an intention, and finding time for sex and romance.

The skills needed for open monogamy relationships:
- Capacity to empathize with our partner
- Insight into our own blind spots
- Ability to articulate our emotions
- Good communication
- Mutual respect
- Finding time for sex and romance

Communicating with Empathy

To build good communication and increase the experience of empathy between you, try this exercise:

The next time you want to talk about something difficult, ask your partner how they feel: "I am curious how you are feeling about _____ right in this moment?" When they share their feelings with you, listen with curiosity and an open mind. Respond with empathy for their feelings. You don't have to agree or explain, just try to understand and relate to how they are feeling. Use these sentence stems:

"I understand that because _____" or "It makes sense that you feel that way because _____" or "You make sense to me because _____."

Then share with them how what they said makes you feel. For instance, "When you say that it makes me feel _____."

This is a good exercise in communicating feelings. It will help you both feel more connected and is a good way to discuss stressful topics. It will serve you well as you formulate your open monogamy agreement.

In chapter 1, Laura and John had just begun their conversation about open monogamy. Laura had asked John if they could reexamine their monogamy. She had met someone through her job and wanted to explore an outside relationship. She was surprised when John agreed right away; he said he wanted her to be happy. In therapy, we began a conversation about what opening their monogamy would look like and I introduced them to the monogamy continuum.

THE MONOGAMY CONTINUUM

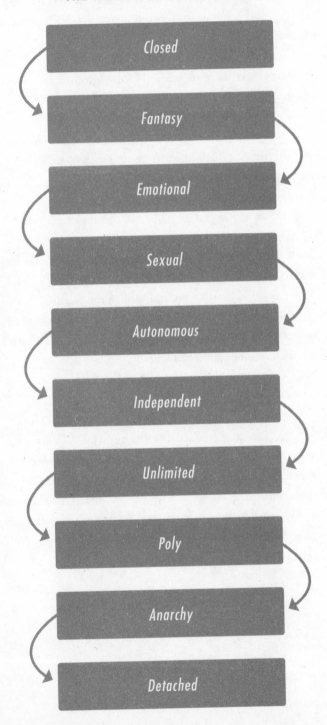

Closed—All sexual and emotional connection stays only between primary partners.

Fantasy—Fantasies of other people (including pornography) do not threaten relationship.

Emotional—Emotional relationships and romantic flirtations are acceptable.

Sexual—Sexual and affectionate play with others, when both are present, is okay.

Autonomous—Open to explore sexual and emotional connections; partner is still top priority.

Independent—Exploring sex with other people with a don't ask, don't tell policy.

Unlimited—Both partners are allowed unlimited sexual or emotional relationships with others.

Poly—Physical, emotional, affectionate, romantic, bonded relationships with multiple partners.

Relationship Anarchy—No hierarchical primary or secondary partners; anything goes.

Detached—One or both partners pull away from partnership and the other must react.

I showed them the options, from totally closed all the way through detaching. I told them they could open their marriage a little or all the way. Laura said, "Right now, my relationship with this other person is still at a *fantasy* place."

I said, "You can integrate that into your monogamy right now. You can agree that it is fine to explore your fantasies about this other person. You can even talk about them with John, if he is okay with it. For some couples, this can be pretty sexy. Other people may find it upsetting. You have to agree first and then do it in a way that is respectful."

John said, "I don't want to know about her fantasies, not about another guy."

Laura said, "I want to take this new relationship to that next level, on that continuum. I want to get to know this person and have some flexibility, and then I want to be more autonomous. I want to have a relationship with them."

"So, you want to move from just fantasy to a more *emotional* exploration of the relationship, and then some kind of *sexual* relationship with this person. This might be through text or by phone? Or do you want to bring this person home and have sex with John there? An *autonomous* open monogamy is where you would be free and open to explore without John being present. But your marriage would still be the priority."

Laura said, "I definitely want our marriage to come first. I guess that means whatever John feels is important. I want to make the decision, though, so I think I want autonomy."

"In order to do that," I said, "you will have to talk openly about what you each want."

John said, "So what you want is to be totally autonomous, to do what you want, see this person, have sex. Do you even want to tell me about it? Can you tell me about it? Do you tell me when you see them? What about after? Should I be telling you what to do here? I have no idea how this works."

Laura said, "I don't know." They both looked at me.

"Let's go through the monogamy continuum, shall we?" They nodded.

"So, the first area of the monogamy continuum is 'totally closed.' We know you don't want to keep the relationship closed; you have both agreed." They both nodded again.

I continued. "Under each area of the monogamy continuum I have a list of questions you can use to begin your discussion, to figure out what you do want. I am going to give you just one question for each area, for now. This can help you start your conversation and narrow down what you want to do."

I told them to read over the questions and answer on a scale of 1 to 5. One means you totally disagree, 5 means you totally agree, and 2 to 4 means you feel somewhere in between. Then I told them they could share their answers in the next session.

"If you want to have the conversation about your monogamy continuum in the next session, I will help you listen to each other, be empathetic, and share your feelings."

They agreed.

John and Laura took these questions home and in the next session discussed their answers and shared their concerns, fears, and excitement as they reflected on their answers. I'll guide you through this same process on page 88.

The key to beginning a new monogamy relationship is to look at the way you structure your relationship currently. You may want to release the old narrative or change it up. What was the old narrative for you? What has monogamy meant to you so far? What do you want it to mean going forward?

Has your relationship been based on traditional monogamy? What part of traditional monogamy would you like to keep? There may be many things that you like in your life and you don't have to give it all up or change everything. Maybe the roles that you and your partner have played up until now have been beneficial for your lifestyle.

Some people believe that married people have more cultural, social, economic, and political advantages than single people. You may enjoy those privileges and not want to give up those benefits by changing your monogamy status. If you are living together and committed, but not married, you may feel the same.

You also might not want to let go of having a monogamous spouse. Having a primary monogamous spouse may give you a sense of security and comfort, and there's nothing wrong with that.

Are there other ideals, standards, or values that are part of traditional monogamy that you want to keep? What values do you align with in your current status? These values do not have to change. You can decide that safety, security, honesty, and commitment are still important. You don't have to change or compromise your values just because you want to open your relationship.

THE IMPORTANCE OF VALUES

Your values are the things you believe in, and they are the foundation of your personal boundaries. *Personal boundaries are self-imposed internalized limits.* Your boundaries are there to help you know when to slow down or back off. They help you grow and can be a way to increase awareness of where you want to grow and expand.

Self-imposed monogamy is based on a set of values that has given you direction and a path to follow, one that has told you the right or wrong way to live. Within the parameters of traditional monogamy some people find comfort. There are values in the ideals of monogamy—they include loyalty, commitment, perseverance, and longevity.

Some values around monogamy can also point in the opposite direction. Those values can feel restrictive, punishing, and shaming. Some of these are old fashioned and outdated, punitive and unconscious. These themes go way back and are often focused on controlling women and meant to prevent and shame women who break their monogamy agreements. (For instance, a seventeenth-century law in Massachusetts said that women would be subjected to the same punishment as witches if they lured men into marriage by wearing high-heeled shoes.)[1]

Monogamy can be a path of shame for both men and women. It can lead to feeling like an outsider if you don't fit into a traditional monogamy relationship configuration. There are many words in our language for those who break the bonds of monogamy. People who don't conform with monogamy can be called a cheater, a freak, a cuckold, a villain, or a slut.

Monogamy is seen less as a continuum and more like a polarity; good or bad, a pass or fail test, a yes or no covenant, a black or white judgment. There has been no room for gray. Not upholding monogamy has been seen as a sign that a person has failed, that they have been weak, not that the relationship agreement has failed or was faulty. The person clearly broke the rules, and the rule breaker's character is now up for review, public evaluation, and scorn.

Monogamy as a continuum flows from totally closed—meaning no sexual, sensual, or emotional connection with others outside of the marriage—to having physical or emotionally affectionate and bonded outside relationships without sex; to having sexual play with others if both partners are present; to totally open, with both partners being allowed to fully explore sexual, sensual, and emotional connections with people beside their primary partner. This can happen while still making that partner the top priority (hence "monogamy") or it can be more like relationship anarchy, where there are no labels or hierarchy, no primary or secondary partners, and everyone is seen as equal. There are no value judgments on the monogamy continuum.

RULES

All romantic and sexual relationships have "rules." Some don't like to call them rules, but rules are basically expectations that are explicitly discussed or implicitly assumed. The rule that marriage includes sex with only one person has variations that might look similar to the monogamy clause but are not necessarily discussed.

For example, some couples consider masturbation private, while others consider it cheating. Others think viewing pornography is a breach of the monogamy rule. In some cases, having a close emotional tie to a friend outside of a relationship can feel like a betrayal, where someone else might go to strip clubs or dance halls and it's not considered a breach.

Other couples have a don't ask, don't tell policy. This can be explicit, where it's agreed that they won't talk about things, or it can be implicitly assumed that as long as it's not discussed, it's not a problem. These types of agreements tend to be "saving face" agreements. To avoid conflict, the couple avoids revealing behaviors to each other that might make their partner feel jealous, hurt, or embarrassed.

Lots of married couples, 25 to 45 percent, claim to be monogamous but are actually involved in *nonconsensual nonmonogamy*, or cheating—a form of nonmonogamy without the partner's consent.[2]

Although on the surface, the relationship may appear to be a traditional marriage, it does not have the exact configuration of monogamy.

For couples with a more transparent agreement, there are still guidelines, but they are more open. Those guidelines can include anything on the monogamy continuum. Monogamy is no longer a one-time choice made at the altar when the couple says "I do." After the "I do," the issue is not closed, never to be discussed again. That's like saying, "I told you I loved you when I married you, so I shouldn't have to ever say it again." Saying "I love you" is not a one-time thing; it doesn't last a lifetime. You have to repeat it often and remind each other that you care. Sharing your love for each other out loud is an important part of staying connected. You need to say "I love you," often. Not because your partner forgets that you love them, but because it means different things under different conditions and at different times throughout a lifetime.

Monogamy is like love. It is an active word, like a verb, rather than a fixed state, a one-time permanent label. To be monogamous, or monogamish, or very monogamous, or less than monogamous, is a choice. Every day one has to choose to actively be committed to whatever type of monogamy fits your relationship. Things may change given the circumstances on any given day.

EXPANSIVE MONOGAMY

You can be very happy and satisfied in every way with your relationship and still want to try an expanded type of monogamy. It's okay to want more. Opening your relationship to other options doesn't in any way mean you love your partner less. It could, in fact, mean you are so comfortable with your partner and your love for each other that you are ready to grow into some exciting, perhaps uncomfortable, and maybe even scary areas.

Even having these conversations could bring new energy to an already exciting partnership. Having a conversation about creating a more fluid relationship means softening all of the boundaries and edges and celebrating what is unique to your version of fidelity. Whatever you decide is entirely up to you.

While we all have fingers, your thumbprint is unique. No one else will ever have your exact thumbprint. Your relationship is like a thumbprint. While everyone you know may have promised some kind of monogamy when they got married, each of their implicit assumptions and the way they demonstrate their monogamy explicitly is expressed in their own inimitable way.

With expansive monogamy you do not have to feel trapped in your coupledom. Your arrangement can grow and stretch with you. As your lives expand, you may share your thoughts and fantasies with each other. You could have a "what if" conversation and talk about things in concept only. You could read erotica out loud to each other or watch erotic films together. You could watch each other masturbate. You could flirt with other couples. You could go out and watch your partner dance with someone else. Or you could have sex with other people when you are together, or when you are apart. Eventually, you might each have full-blown sexual experiences in an unlimited way, or a polyamorous relationship, which would include other love relationships in your marriage.

Your arrangement could contract during times when you want your monogamy to be just between the two of you. It might change or shift when you need a rest or a break, or you need more attention or time. There is no one path to create your coupledom. You are exceptional, you are a rare team, and you can create your dream life together; one that works for you.

BEGINNING THE UNCOMFORTABLE CONVERSATION

You could skip to chapter 7 and jump right into finding your place on the monogamy continuum, but not every couple is ready for that. To begin the conversation, think about how comfortable you are discussing open monogamy. Will you feel awkward? Are you worried it will make your partner uncomfortable? What if you aren't sure how to bring up any of these things? What if you don't even know what you want?

It's okay if you don't know exactly what you want your new open monogamy to look like. It's okay to just be curious about what expanded monogamy could be like between you. There are three categories of interest that most people fall into when thinking about opening their monogamous relationship.

Curious

If you are interested in making your boundaries a little more fluid, maybe talking about how other people do it, reading books about it, or asking a therapist or coach about open monogamy, you may be curious. You might find yourself "tuning in" to things you hear about or experiences that are new to you, things that you want to learn more about. These tune ins are not necessarily things you fantasize about, nor are they situations that you want to move on, yet. You could be just fine with the way things are now and in no rush to change anything.

If that's the case, you can tell your partner, *"I'm curious about how people open their marriage, I wonder how they make it work. I wonder if we know anyone who does it and if we could we talk with them?"* Or, *"I have read this book and I am hoping you and I could read parts of it together?"*

Being curious about something doesn't mean you ever have to do it. You may be in the learning phase of your exploration and want to discover what this is all about and think carefully through your options. You might decide you never want to change your current agreement and that everything is fine the way it is. Share those feelings with your partner if that's the way you feel. Sometimes just being curious about something and talking about it is a way to bond and can bring a heightened level of excitement to your intimate lives.

Fantasy/Turn Ons

You may be more than curious. You may have thoughts about opening your monogamy, and thinking about those things may turn you on. You may have a desire to know more about these turn ons. They are exciting, and you find you are thinking about them more often.

You can have fantasies of what something would be like and still not be quite ready to do anything about it. Sharing your fantasies with your partner can be difficult.

Usually, our fantasies are our own private, internal domain. Sometimes we don't want to share a fantasy if we don't really want to act it out or aren't quite ready to make it come true. We could be hesitant to share our fantasies with our partner because we worry they could be more ready than we are to take things to the next level.

It's okay to let your partner know you just want to talk about your fantasies before you ever put them into action. You might want to say to them, *"I have been fantasizing about what an open relationship would look like. Sometimes I think about certain things and they are a turn on for me. I am a little hesitant to talk about this because I don't want you to think I'm ready to do anything, not right away, and maybe not ever. But I would like to share my fantasies with you. Is that okay?"*

Having fantasies about what it would be like is the first step to a more open conversation with your partner. They may have similar fantasies, or they could be quite different. They may have never thought about any of this and be quite shocked that you are bringing it up at all. It can be helpful to reassure them that this is still a fantasy for you. Let them know you want to do this as a couple and you look forward to having lots of conversations before anything happens.

Action

You may have already thought about opening your monogamy and you want to do it now. It's time, you think, the perfect time, to expand the boundaries of your relationship and start taking some risks. It's time to take on some of your fantasies. These could include, for instance, adding other people or sexual experiences into your lives.

The best way to bring this up to your partner is to be honest. Tell them, *"I've been reading up on open monogamy. One thing that seems interesting to me and might be hot for us to do is _____. I think this could be really fun for us. Would you like to know more about what I'm proposing?"*

Keep in mind that you may be in a different place than your partner. They may not be ready to take on this fantasy or take the next step. They may need to talk about things for a while, review the details, talk about their feelings, and understand more about what this means for your relationship.

In a later chapter we will review how to discuss your expectations and your own redlines and requests in order to formulate a clear agreement each time you want to push the edge of your monogamy. Even if you are not ready to talk to your partner, try this exercise to clarify what actual actions you might want to take and what is simply fun to imagine.

Fantasy Scale

Are you curious? Is this a fantasy? Or are you ready to take this into action? Ask yourself the following questions, fill in the blank with whatever you are imagining, and rate it on a scale of 1 to 5:

1 not really true

2 somewhat true

3 kind of true

4 very true

5 totally true

Curious:

I am curious about _____ and wonder how people do it. **1 2 3 4 5**

I wonder if I know anyone who does _____. **1 2 3 4 5**

I want to talk with someone who does _____ to see how they do _____. **1 2 3 4 5**

I have read about _____ or seen ____ on the internet. **1 2 3 4 5**

I want to explore _____ more with you or on my own. **1 2 3 4 5**

Fantasy:

I have been fantasizing about what
___ would look like. 1 2 3 4 5

I think about ___ and it is a turn on for me. 1 2 3 4 5

I am not ready to do anything right now,
but I like imagining ___. 1 2 3 4 5

I am not sure I ever want to ___, but
it is a possibility. 1 2 3 4 5

I would like to share my fantasies
about ___ with you. 1 2 3 4 5

Action:

I've been planning how to ___ for a while. 1 2 3 4 5

I think ___ would be hot/interesting/good
for us and we should do it. 1 2 3 4 5

I propose that we ___ as soon as possible. 1 2 3 4 5

I have imagined the steps to make
___ happen. 1 2 3 4 5

I have a clear plan and want to
implement ___ soon. 1 2 3 4 5

The higher your score on the fantasy scale, the more likely
you are ready to put your plan into action.

○

HOW DO YOU KNOW YOU'RE READY?

Once you are talking about your fantasies, you are discussing things that turn you on and sharing what might be hot for you. When you have discussed some of your most personal thoughts, you may already be seeing the possibilities and be moving beyond being simply curious. You have begun experiencing the ways open monogamy could work for you. You may already feel more expansive. This could be a sign you are ready to explore and take things into action.

When is the right time to begin? How do you know you are both really ready to start? Are there signs, things you should notice that are indicators that now is the right time?

WHAT-IFS

It might be a sign you are ready for more if you find you are talking about the "what ifs." The what-if conversations are discussions about the potential for action; all of the crazy, sexy ideas you have of being with other people. When both of you are curious, or having fantasies about what it might be like to expand things, you might be ready to move from just talking about things to real action. Being ready to take on a real scenario is risky, but you can test it out first by asking a lot of what-ifs.

You may have talked about having sex with other people—maybe a threesome with someone you know or perhaps one of you has a friend who you want to explore something more with but aren't sure how to do it. You might have talked about it and both feel fine with it and there are no hard feelings, neither of you feel coerced or manipulated, and you are both turned on by the thought. Talking about and fantasizing about these experiences before you have them could be a sign you want to move to the next level.

Keep in mind this is not a definite sign. Sometimes just talking about these possibilities can be enough. It can be exciting and stimulating to have discussions about these kinds of fantasies. But, if you find you are sharing your fantasies often, talking about what you would be doing and what they would be doing and who would be doing what to whom and where and what everyone would be wearing, then you might be ready.

Before you take things into action, consider the potential emotional consequences of your actions. A what-if conversation can help.

PAUL AND JACK

Paul and Jack had been in therapy for a year, struggling with their mutual lack of interest in sex. They once had a full and erotic life together, but lately it had gone downhill for both of them.

One day in our session we began a what-if discussion. Nothing had ever happened outside of their marriage, but they been talking about finding something to spice things up.

Paul brought it up first. "I've been wondering if you have ever thought about us having sex with other people?"

Jack looked at him and laughed. "Are you bringing this up in therapy because you are afraid of what I'd say when you asked me this?"

Paul hesitated. "Yes, kind of. But I want you to know I am only feeling curious about this. As two gay men, it seems like we should want to do this. Our friends all have open relationships and you and I have been monogamous for twenty years."

Jack said, "I can't say I have never thought about it. Have you?"

Paul said, "I have always been curious about it, but you and I have never talked about it so I guess I was afraid of what you would think if I brought it up."

I suggested they go home and talk about this using a what-if conversation.

"Talk about what each of you might find exciting if you were to open your marriage. Just discuss anything you might be curious about right now," I said. "You don't have to do anything, not yet, or ever, but talk about the things that might interest you."

The what-if conversation is a way to talk about fantasies you might be wondering about, and check those things out with your partner. Are they hot for you? Are they exciting? Are they a turn on? Should we ever try these things? Are they okay to talk about? It doesn't mean you have to do any of those things; you're just talking about them for now.

"What if some of the things we talk about are a turn on?" asked Paul. "Does that mean we share that with each other? What if the other person gets mad or upset?"

I said, "You might be turned on by talking about these things, but a turn on is not necessarily a take on. A take on is when you actually take on a fantasy. You bring it into action, you agree to do something, and you make it happen. Just talking about these things doesn't mean you want to do them. The idea is to talk about what's hot for you. Just this kind of conversation can bring some erotic energy back into your relationship."

"We do need some more erotic energy," Jack said. Paul agreed.

Here are some of examples of the what-ifs Paul and Jack discussed at home:

What if we slept in separate bedrooms?

What if we tried something different during sex?

What if we kissed other people in front of each other?

What if we went to a sex club and just watched?

What if we were naked together with someone else?

What if we had a threesome with one of our friends?

What if you had sex with a sex worker in front of me?

What if we added a third person, a love partner, in our relationship?

Using your own ideas, create a list of what-ifs and take turns with your partner, asking them what-if. You can both answer in a way that reflects how much you would like it, or not like it, or how sexy it sounds to you, or how uncomfortable it makes you.

Before you agree to shifting any of these what-ifs into an action, both of you need to discuss, agree, and consent.

DISCUSS

Before turning a fantasy into action, discuss in detail exactly what you want to do. This conversation can include a detailed description of who will do what and where and to whom.

You may want to start with something where no one does anything to anyone, yet. You could try something voyeuristic, like going to a sex club or a sex party. Destination vacations, swinger clubs, and sex clubs allow beginners to check out the scene without participating. You can walk around and observe people having sex, or you can join in if you feel motivated. There are clubs in most cities and you can find parties through Meetup groups online.

If you agree that this is a good place to start, have a discussion to set up the ground rules and expectations. What is your interest in this event? What are your requests and what are your redlines? Do you want to watch or participate? If you want to participate, what type of participation is ideal for you? What if you change your mind when you get there? How do you talk about that in the moment? Where do you see yourself at the end of the night? Will you stay together throughout the experience, or is it okay to explore separately and meet up at the end of the night?

AGREE

Research shows that people assume men are the ones who pressure women into open relationships, when in fact, it's women who tend to be the gatekeepers of open monogamy. If an open relationship happens, it's usually because the woman says it's okay and agrees to it.

But it can be hard to agree on everything. It doesn't matter if you are a man or a woman, gay or straight, what you will try, how things will go, and who makes the final decisions can vary.

One way to find a place of agreement is to search for experiences that could be mutually pleasurable. Both of you should want to do them and like the idea. You may feel differently about it when you get there, but you should agree on the basic idea of the act or the outing.

It's easier to agree on things before you get there and before anyone takes their clothes off. It can be difficult to try and stop things once you have begun. You might be embarrassed or afraid you will upset your partner if you try to call things off.

In their what-if conversation, Paul and Jack talked about their fantasies of going to a sex club. They wanted to at least watch other people and see what it would look like to be around other gay couples having sex. They were both turned on thinking about sex happening in a public place.

They found a dance club that looked, from the website, like it could lead to a hot, sexy night. Before they went to the club, they discussed it and agreed on a few things. One, that neither of them would leave the other person's side throughout the night, which was a request of Jack's. Two, if they did meet another man or a couple of men, the most either would do was kiss, which was Paul's request. And three, they agreed that if either of them felt awkward at all, they would leave at the first sign of discomfort from either of them. This was a redline for both of them. Neither Paul nor Jack wanted to feel that they were staying if their partner felt uncomfortable.

Safe Words

Before going to the club, Paul and Jack came in for a session to discuss their feelings and their fears. They were worried that they wouldn't be able to recognize when their partner was uncomfortable and were concerned that one of them could be having a good time while the other was miserable.

I suggested they come up with a *safe word*. A safe word is a code word they would both agree on that, regardless of what was happening in the evening, would indicate that one of them was uncomfortable and would mean that they would both need to immediately leave the club, no questions asked. Using a safe word was a redline boundary for both of them, one they agreed to comply with no matter what. A redline cannot be crossed.

"A safe word can help you feel like you are together in this but you also have your own personal space," I said.

"What if I'm not sure I want to leave but something happens that freaks you out?" Paul said.

"You can have two safe words, one that means, 'Hey, we need to talk and evaluate what is happening, but not necessarily leave right in this moment.' The other safe word can be the hard redline word for 'Let's get out of here now, no questions asked,'" I said.

Paul said, "That could work for us; we can check in with each other throughout the night and see if the safe word thing is necessary."

I explained, "For instance, your first safe word could be 'orange' and your second safe word could be 'red.' This is like a secret code. The word 'orange' means you need to slow down, take a break, and talk about what's happening. If you use the safe word 'red,' it means for whatever reason, the whole thing is too much and one of you is saying, 'we have to leave.' You both have to agree on this ahead of time."

Jack said, "We definitely need to agree. We both have to abide by the safe words, no matter what."

Paul said, "I agree!"

They talked about what might happen at the club.

Paul said, "What if things get exciting and we want to, you know, play with someone? More than kissing."

I asked Jack, "When do you want Paul to check in with you? When he feels like he wants to play with someone, kiss someone, take his clothes off? Can we get specific here?"

Jack said, "I guess I would have to assess the situation when we are there."

CONSENT

Consent means you give your partner the green light to do something to you or someone else or to have something done to you. Consent should be verbal, clear, and obvious. If one partner wants to add something to the relationship, the other partner should express their consent or permission for that to happen. This is important in all aspects of your monogamy agreement, but especially when agreeing to anything that has to do with physical or sexual boundaries.

There is a difference between implied and expressed consent. In this case, it is important to verbally express consent. Implied consent means the other person assumes you give consent based on your actions or lack of action. For instance, not disagreeing or not stopping an action is considered implied consent. So much could go wrong with implied consent. Too many actions or nonactions can be misinterpreted, so implied consent should never be used as consent.

Consent should always be expressed and informed. In other words, you should know what you are getting into. It is hard to consent to something you know nothing about. For instance, you cannot give informed consent to a sexual experience in a club ahead of time if you have never been to a club and have no idea what could happen there. You may need to wait and see what happens when you get there and give consent in the moment.

The consent should be mutual. Mutual consent is when you both agree to something. Mutual consent should be enthusiastic and positive. You should not feel pressure to consent. You should feel informed and excited to consent.

Excited, informed, and mutually expressed consent makes anything you are doing more fun and safer for everyone involved. It is the opposite of badgering or bugging or pushing or cajoling. You shouldn't need to wheedle or beg. You shouldn't have to persuade your partner to let go of their own boundaries and values. It's not consent if you have to wear someone down until they give in.

Consent should be given freely and joyfully. If it's given somewhat hesitantly, that can be okay, but check in with your partner. Most of us are not 100 percent sure of anything until we try it. Talk about it and be sure they know what they are consenting to and all is clear.

ALWAYS CONSENT, NEVER COERCION

You should never feel coerced, forced, or pressured in any way to swing, have sex, or be in an open relationship of any kind.

If you aren't 100 percent in, then don't do it. You might not be ready. Talk about any hesitation with your partner. Talk about why you aren't ready or what you might not want to do and why.

It's better to talk now about any concerns to prevent feeling resentment later. In a later chapter we will talk about how to *pre-vent* by discussing problems before they become real conflicts. If you don't consent to an act, speak up now before you do something against your will.

There are many reasons why a partner might try to coerce you into an open monogamy agreement. Sometimes a partner may pressure you into nonmonogamy because they are ready to take something into action and you might still be at the curiosity stage. Or, it may be that they are getting impatient with the process because they have been thinking about this for much longer than you have.

Both of you should consent to whatever it is you want to try. You may have different interest levels, and you might be operating at different speeds. You might be more or less eager than your partner to begin. But you should never feel pressured into anything, nor should you pressure or bully your spouse into taking a fantasy into action. You don't have to both have the same turn on in order to take on a fantasy, but you should both wholeheartedly consent to it.

If you feel like you are being pressured into anything in your open monogamy, don't do it. You should never enter an open relationship because you feel guilty or are trying to please your partner if, in fact, you don't want to do it. You should always feel like you give consent without coercion.

True consent is always consensual. If you feel pressured or bullied into giving in to the arrangement, you will eventually resent it and resent your partner and your whole relationship is bound to collapse. When you truly consent to something it means you can say "hell yes" and you can also change your mind. Consent is an active thing; it lives and breathes as your relationship changes and grows.

3 Ps of Consent

Use this dialogue to start a conversation about potential possibilities, problems, and positives before you consent:

What are the potential issues that could arise if I consent to this?

Make a list of the possibilities and list any problems that could come up as well as any positives. See if you can make a list of ten problems and ten positives for each possibility.

Possibilities	Problems	Positives

Now, read through your list.

Do the possibilities, problems, and positives make sense? Are they realistic? Does one possibility look more problematic or positive than another?

Now, challenge your own narratives. How realistic are each of these possibilities, problems, and positives? Keep in mind that just because you wrote these down doesn't mean any of these possibilities has to happen nor do the problems have to occur.

Can you share your list with your partner?

Here is an example of three things Paul and Jack discussed using Paul's list.

Possibilities	Problems	Positives
We go to the sex club	I don't like it	I like it
We have a great time	You want to go back	You start feeling sexy again
We meet another guy	I get jealous	I feel interested and sexy

This type of list is a way to begin a dialogue, communicating and getting comfortable with sharing your feelings. The goal is to talk about your concerns before consenting to anything. When sharing the list, both partners want to feel heard and have their feelings validated.

Sharing the list can be tough. You can read it out loud, or if you've written it down, you can let your partner read it. Have your partner empathize with what you've written and try to avoid explaining or giving advice. Instead, use empathic statements like, "It makes sense you feel that way because ____."

If your partner don't seem to be responding with active listening, you can ask for empathy. Asking for empathy would sound like, "Can you tell me what makes sense to you about what I have on my list? You don't have to agree or disagree, or promise or explain, just let me know you understand my feelings."

When you have had a thorough discussion about the possibilities, the potential problems, and the positives, ask your partner to share their list with you. Empathize with them about their feelings.

After you have both shared and you both feel heard, decide what possibilities you can consent to with a strong feeling of pleasure. Consent should feel like a very hot "yes" based on the limited information you have. This does not mean you are ready to take the possibility into action; it just means that you are feeling out the hot yes potential and sharing that with your partner.

When Paul shared his list in our session, I helped both of them work on empathy. Jack responded to Paul's potential problem about being jealous by saying, "It makes sense that you might be afraid we will meet another guy. That makes perfect sense. We are both handsome men, of course the guys in that club will want us. We might be old," he laughed, "but we're not dead yet."

"Nice empathy," I said. "Can you validate Paul's feelings about his fear of jealousy?"

Jack said, "It makes sense that you are afraid you'll feel jealous. You do worry that I will want to be with someone else. I don't want anyone else, don't worry about that."

"What should he do that night if you are talking to someone and he feels jealous?" I asked.

Jack looked at Paul. "You can talk to me and use the safe word if you want to leave. But tell me, is that what you want? Should I not talk to anyone? What do you want?" Jack sounded annoyed.

"Empathy means you try and understand how he feels," I said.

"I understand, but it makes me anxious to think he might get freaked out at the club," Jack said.

Paul said, "It makes sense that you are afraid that I will freak out. I do get jealous. But I am also intrigued by the whole thing. I don't mind feeling a little bit jealous, but if it makes me really crazy, I am pulling the safe word for sure."

I asked, "What can you consent to, both of you?"

Jack said, "I consent to a hot yes, to meeting other guys. We can talk to other people; I am all for that if Paul is okay with it. And I promise I am not interested in leaving with anyone."

Paul said, "I am okay with that too. Maybe not quite as much of a hot yes. But I can give my full consent right now. Let's go and have a good time and talk to whoever we want."

Consent on both sides is the most important step. Once you both agree, you are well on your way.

CHAPTER FIVE

Navigating Different Needs

In my office, Frederika sat with her arms wrapped tight around her waist. Her long red hair glowed in the morning light that was streaming in through my office window.

"No matter what I do for Pierre, it will never be enough. I have tried to be a good partner and have given him every sexual thing he has asked for, but there is always more he wants. I am not good enough for him; he will always want someone else."

Pierre, a tall thin man wearing an impeccably tailored suit, sat stiffly at the edge of his chair. "Frederika, of course you are good enough. You are wonderful. I love our life together."

"Then why do you want someone else?" she cried. "If I was good enough for you, this would not be an issue."

We all have stories we tell ourselves, thoughts or schemas that are organized around narratives we have been telling ourselves our whole lives, some good, some not so positive. They live inside of us, patterns of thinking that we slip into in times of stress. They are ways of thinking that our mind uses to organize our experiences and explain our world. It is a filing system to explain our past, present, and future. But these schemas or stories may not be based on reality. Some schemas are narratives that are, instead, a reflection of our self-esteem or lack of self-confidence. Patterns of thought that reflect low self-worth and feelings of shame can surface when we have relationship stress. Old messages we have internalized can emerge, like not being good enough or not deserving happiness.

Frederika's narrative, her internal thoughts, seemed to circle around a story that she is less than. That narrative was triggered by Pierre asking for something outside of their monogamy.

Pierre insisted it had nothing to do with her not being good enough. He wanted something that he could not ask her for. And he preferred to seek it outside of their marriage, to compartmentalize it, and keep it separate from their sexual relationship. Frederika believed that Pierre wanted to open their marriage because she could not be everything for him. This activated old feelings she had since childhood.

In therapy, we worked on two goals. First, the goal was to help Pierre express his needs clearly, so that Frederika could understand what he wanted. And the second goal was to help Frederika let go of the past and to know that Pierre's needs did not mean she was deficient.

I asked Pierre to be clear with Frederika about what he wanted.

"Are you curious about this, is this a fantasy, or are you ready to take this into action?" I asked. "Curious would mean you are just sort of wondering about what it would be like; maybe you've been doing some research or looking it up on the internet. Fantasy would mean this is really exciting for you. It might be something you've been thinking about and getting turned on by for a while. It may be the only way you get turned on, and you've never shared it, or it could be a new fantasy. Or you could be ready to do this, whatever it is. You might want to take this into action. Maybe you've already planned it out. Maybe you've met someone. Maybe you've already begun. Let's start the conversation and see where you are on this scale of curiosity/fantasy/action."

Pierre did the fantasy scale and marked down a five on every measure. "I am ready," he said. "This is not just something I am curious about, nor is it just a fantasy. I have been thinking about this for a long, long time."

"Can you tell her more about this, Pierre?" I asked. "The next step here is to discuss and communicate. Let's talk about what it is you are thinking about and then let's talk about the possibilities."

Pierre hesitated and finally said, "I have always wondered what it would be like to explore a kink relationship. Frederika, you and I have tried to talk about this in the past. I know you are not comfortable with it. I don't want to pressure you into doing something you are not into."

Frederika sat quietly for a moment. "Does this mean you would be with another woman?"

"Yes, I want to be with a dom, a dominant."

A *dom* or *dominant* is someone who, in a BDSM relationship, would take charge of a role-play scenario, acting out the part of the initiator and taking on the more aggressive part in a bondage, domination, sadomasochism fantasy. Pierre explained that he had these BDSM fantasies all of his life, but that he knew Frederika was not turned on by them. He wanted to act them out for once in his life, and outsourcing them to another partner seemed to be a way to protect her from these desires and give him a way to explore his fantasies with someone who could meet his needs.

"I am not comfortable with you being with someone else, not yet. I don't think so, I am not sure now, we need to discuss this further," Frederika said.

Pierre said, "I don't want to lie to you. I don't want to do this behind your back. Not ever. I will only do this if you are open to the idea and we agree on everything."

Frederika thought about it and looked at him. "What would it mean for me? What would I do?"

He said, "You could explore with someone as well. I would find someone, a female dominant, and have a session with her, with your permission of course. If you want to have a date with someone, anyone, it is okay with me. I would want each of us to do this separately, privately, without the other one present. I feel I personally need to do this on my own."

Frederika took a deep breath. "I don't know how to go from here," she said.

I said, "The next steps are to discuss the possibilities, the potential problems, and the ways this could potentially be good for your relationship, and come to an agreement if you can."

I told them about the 3 Ps. Listing all the potential possibilities, problems, and positives can make the conversation feel manageable when the feelings become overwhelming.

I asked them both to make a list of their potential possibilities, problems, and positives.

When they came back for the next session, Pierre brought in his list. Frederika was crying when she read it out loud.

"I am afraid," she said, "that what you want is wrong, and if you do this, I will somehow be giving you permission."

Possibilities	Problems	Positives
Find a dominant	Privacy, finances	It might be easy?
Have a session	I might not like it	I could love it
Tell Fred	She might end our marriage	Fred could have her own session

I asked Pierre if he could empathize with her, even though he was very upset. We had been practicing empathy, so he knew he could start with a "It makes sense you feel that way" statement.

"Frederika, it makes sense, knowing about your very strict religious childhood that you might think that anything outside of a traditional, vanilla-type of sex is dirty. When you say that, it hurts me deeply. I also don't need your permission. But I would like to do this with consent and with your agreement. I would not want to do this behind your back."

"Vanilla sex" refers to sex that is traditional, hetero-focused, and usually includes *penis-in-vagina intercourse (PIV)*.

"But it's wrong!" she said. "There must be something wrong with me. I am not enough for you. Our sex is not enough for you. If our sex life was enough for you, you wouldn't need this."

I asked Frederika to stop and think about what she was feeling. "Notice what is happening in your body, what you are experiencing, what emotions are coming up for you."

"I know this comes from my childhood, but I cannot stop these feelings," .e od... .. s lliy ..l.

"What if this was no one's fault? What if there was nothing wrong with you, or with Pierre?" I asked

"But I don't want to be a dominant for him," she said. "I cannot do this for him."

"" ....1 ..:1 "т ..... ro make you do it if you don't want

Pierre did not want Frederika to pretend to like something if it was a turnoff for her. "We have a wonderful sexual life. You give me everything I want, except for this."

This was not about him feeling something was lacking in their relationship, but rather a desire to expand on what they already had. I asked Frederika to say more about her fear of not being enough for Pierre.

"If I was enough sexually and emotionally he wouldn't have to look outside of our marriage," she said.

I asked Pierre, "What does it feel like when she says this?"

He said, "I love her. I do want more, but *I want more of me*. It's not because she is not enough. I am craving a different side of myself. I want to grow into something else, to experiment, to expand."

Frederika said, "I understand. I do. I don't want to stop you. I want to only support you to grow, you know that."

"I do know that."

She said, quietly, "I am also attracted to the idea of discovering more of myself, to be honest. I don't want to be in a kinky relationship, but I do wonder who I would be if I were with someone else. I have thought about it, of course. To be with someone I wasn't married to, who doesn't see me as a wife or the mother of their child, this could be interesting for me, perhaps."

FEAR-BASED MONOGAMY

For Frederika and Pierre, as with any relationship, opening your monogamy should not be coercive, or based on the idea that if you say "no" your partner will break up with you, cheat on you, or hold it against you. Entering into open monogamy because you feel held hostage by your partner's emotional needs can only make things complicated at best and abusive at worst.

Your monogamy should never be based on fear. If you are staying in a traditional monogamy relationship because you are afraid of opening up, but inside, you really want a more flexible relationship, you may be living in fear. It can be hard to tell your partner what you want, but telling them the truth

Some people are afraid to tell their partner their real desires for fear their partner will leave. If you tell your partner you want a more open relationship, what will they say? Your concerns may be based more on the fact that you don't know how to talk to them and less on the fact that they will get angry and leave you. You may need more and better language to ask you for what you want.

Trying to fix a relationship with an open relationship is like trying to mend the broken foundation of a house by adding more weight on top. If you are in a strained relationship, or one suffering from betrayal after an affair, trying to negotiate an additional relationship and more partners is only going to add more stress. You will need to mend the relationship you have first, or else you risk the whole structure coming down around you.

Open relationships require maturity and maintenance. The deep and constant level of communication required is not what most people are taught in their families of origin and certainly not in school. It will take a great investment of time, energy, and possibly therapy to learn the empathy, validation, and compassion needed to listen to your partner and what they want and need. It also takes skills to understand your own emotions and be able to soothe yourself when things go wrong.

PASSION

During my thirty years as a therapist, I have seen thousands of couples. I can predict with a certain level of therapeutic accuracy where couples are in their intimacy based on their conversations around monogamy. It is clear that when a committed partnership gets to a certain point, one or both partners often report a loss of passion in their relationship. They will begin to question whether a new relationship could restore their personal feeling of aliveness. Some fantasize about falling in love again and some begin to search for a new love or new relationship energy. There are ways to avoid this seemingly inevitable marriage expiration date that so many couples experience. And it is possible to do this without opening your relationship. Many people stay together after these challenging turning points in a marriage and find even more passion than ever before.

Using an open marriage to try to wake up your current marriage is a fine idea, only if you both agree that you are doing it to bring erotic energy into your sex life. As you may have noticed from the couples profiled so far, it can be a lot of work and added stress to have these conversations, and it's not as sexy as you might imagine.

Here is an exercise to remind you to play and enjoy each other right now.

Talk and Play

The following questions can help you create more play and aliveness in your relationship. You can each repeat back what you hear, mirroring and validating one another's answers. There's no need to take anything into action. Just have fun with it. Listen, share, and enjoy.

Write your answers down or share them out loud with your partner. Have your partner share their answers with you:

What is something you like about our relationship?

What is something you feel we do well together?

What is the most fun you and I have ever had together?

What is something you would love to repeat in our life?

Can you tell me one part of my body you totally adore?

What is one thing you appreciate about our sex life?

What is one thing you like about your own body?

What is something I do that makes you feel sexy?

If you could sleep with any movie or TV star, who would it be?

What is your favorite sexual position?

If there had to be a pet name for each of us, what would they be?

What is one thing you like about yourself?

Can you roll your tongue or do
something weird with your body?

What was the most exciting moment
of your entire life?

What is one thing you are truly grateful for?

DON'T FORGET TO PLAY

What is play and why do we need it? According to Nan Wise, a neu-
rologist, researcher, and sex therapist, play is the joyful occupation of
all young mammals. Play is how we all learn as children. We learn to
explore the world, our bodies, and our senses through play. We play to
experiment, with ourselves and other people. Play teaches us how to
socialize. It's a natural way to rehearse the important skills needed to be
a grown-up. The adult skills necessary to survive and thrive start with
imitating our adult caretakers and playing, turning what looks serious
into practice, and having fun with it.

Wise said, "Mammals learn all of the skills necessary for everything from
hunting to foraging for food, to courtship and mating though play. Play is
how we learn to get along with others, whether we are competing, cooper-
ating, engaging, wooing, and mating—and how we learn who is safe, and
who should be avoided in such pursuits."

She said that when our play system is in balance, we have a good sense of
humor, we know how to relax, and we know how to have fun and amuse
ourselves. Sex is part of that play system, as adults.

It's why we call sex toys, "toys." Adults can take sex way too seriously and
put a lot of pressure on themselves and on their partners.

Those who can be in an open monogamy relationship and enjoy their
sexual pursuits, playing with others for the pure joy of interacting, find they
have fewer stressful conversations, fewer moments of jealousy, and they can
take themselves and their situations less seriously with fewer problematic
expectations. As adults, play can help us reduce stress and help us handle

Opening your marriage may require difficult conversations that can trigger fears of abandonment. Maintaining your connection through enjoyment and play can help you stay connected and positive as you make your way through these potentially tough times.

IS THIS A NEGOTIATION?

Some couples like the idea of rules; others don't like rules at all. You can call them rules, or suggestions, or whatever you want. *But keep in mind, rules are meant to control people*. Rules are by nature, constraints. Rules are something a parent instills in a child, a teacher imposes on a student, or a government enforces on a citizen. We, as humans, respond to rules by feeling restricted. Rules are meant to be broken. The whole point of open monogamy is to not feel limited.

Negotiating can also be problematic. Negotiating feels like bargaining, a way to work with the rules. If you tend toward a more anarchist model of open relationship, you aren't going to want anyone telling you what you can or cannot do. If you want a more egalitarian relationship, you will balk at your partner trying to control your behaviors by setting down procedures, negotiating their way into a policy with which you must comply. By telling you what you can or cannot do, or how you should or shouldn't behave, they are creating a controlling, parentified relationship.

Negotiating implies that there will be a winner and a loser. You will have to work to get what you want in the negotiation, and someone will lose some of what is important to them. The partner with the best arbitration skills, the one who is the most articulate or who bargains with the best oratory talent will most likely get more of what they desire and the partner who tends to be more of a pleaser, or is more conflict avoidant, will tend to give in, letting go of their own needs and feeling resentful in the end. Negotiation for an open agreement can be conflictual.

COMPROMISE

Compromising means no one wins and someone always loses. Most likely both of you will have to give up some of what you want. The feeling of having to give up something that is important to you, or having to compromise one's own boundaries, can make what you are agreeing to feel nonconsensual.

BOUNDARIES

Instead of rules or negotiation or compromise, think instead of setting your own personal boundaries. Boundaries are flexible and more subjective than rules. Boundaries are your own experience of the world, and delineate what you need to feel safe, creating freedom within which you can explore.

In fact, one-third (39 percent) of people in polyamorous relationships are resistant to terms like "allow," "restrict," or "rules" because they signify one partner having control over the other. An open monogamy should give you a feeling of freedom, not anxiety.

In the early stages of exploring open monogamy, you will go through a romantic stage similar to being in a new relationship, where you will be breaking through your own boundaries, and you might feel an unlimited new freedom. This comes from stretching the boundaries of old societal restrictions and breaking out of traditional monogamy. When you break free of old sex roles and stereotypes you might feel uninhibited and unrestrained for the first time.

The adventure of discovering sexual freedom can lead to even greater exploration and more personal autonomy in the world. You may heal from things in your past, like old narratives around shame. Old traumas can be resolved. By pushing your boundaries into new situations and relationships and letting down your guard, emotionally and psychologically, you may find you change those inner schemas and stories and see fundamental changes in your personality.

PROMISES

Something to think about when you're creating a new agreement is that it is important not to just make promises. Remember, you may have made promises when you got married or pledged your fidelity.

A promise, any promise, is only as good as the people who promise it. If you agree to something and one person feels absolutely strong in their commitment to the promise, they can feel betrayed if the other person is not as strong in their commitment or belief in the promise. The other partner may believe in the relationship, in their love for the partner, and in a new form of promise, but they may not believe that the promise applies any longer. This in no way means that they are not committed to the relationship.

Your relationship may not be the problem; it may be the promise that is the problem. The promise may be outdated and may no longer apply to the relationship you are living today. I'll give you an example, although some of you may not like this example at all. For vegans: trigger warning.

For ten years, from the time I was 23 to 33, I was a vegetarian. I didn't drink and I didn't do drugs. I felt clean. I did yoga, I took walks, I took up jogging. I went to therapy and I learned to meditate. I didn't eat red meat. It wasn't for any particular reason that I gave up red meat, but once I did it, I made a promise to myself that I would be meat-free, occasionally eating fish or chicken, but no beef, pork, or any other red flesh.

That promise worked for me at the time. It was a promise I made to myself. I felt good about it. When the opportunity to eat meat came up, I remembered my promise and stayed true to it. Some days were harder than others. I held onto the integrity of my meat-free existence.

Then I got pregnant. When I was pregnant with my son, one day, in my first trimester, my body screamed, "Give me a cheeseburger!" It was all I thought about. Meat. Red meat. I wanted a thick, juicy cheeseburger, cooked on a grill. I dreamt about cheeseburgers. Finally, I decided that it was time to change the promise I made to myself and I ate the first cheeseburger I had eaten in ten years. It was the best thing I ever tasted. After that, I ate a steak. I gave my body what it needed.

My promise, the promise I had made to myself, had evolved. I wasn't *breaking* my promise to myself, I didn't feel that I had let myself down, or that things were falling apart. My relationship to food and my commitment to be-

g meat-free was not the problem, nor was my wavering stance on vegetarianism. It was simply that the promise I had made ten years ago, when I was child free and in a different time of my life, in a different body, with different needs, no longer applied to the relationship with myself that I was living that day.

Now, for you, a new agreement is required and should include new rules.

Built in to this new agreement will be ways to create fluidity and variety

SELF-DISCOVERY—FREDERIKA AND PIERRE

"I'm attracted to the discovery of myself," said Frederika, who was still having trouble wrapping her mind around Pierre's desire to be with a sexual dominant, and the couple were still in therapy to work on their open marriage. Frederika was forty-two years old, the CEO of her own corporation, and the mother of two young children, a boy, eight, and a girl, fourteen. Pierre had been a stay-at-home dad throughout their marriage. He was a bilingual musician and made his living giving lessons to French students. In the fourth session, Pierre said, "I love you, I don't want a divorce, and I don't want to have an affair. But I still have these interests."

Frederika looked at him. "I'm still hurt that you want to be with a dominant."

He said, "I have these alternative interests" and looked at her shyly.

I encouraged him to go on. "It can be scary at first to share your interests if you've never talked about them before," I said, "but if you've thought about these things enough to be talking now about opening your marriage, it's important."

Pierre said, "I want you to listen and be open. This is not about me wanting a girlfriend. I want to try some things and I am quite sure you do not like kinky things. I am sure of that."

Frederika said, "I am hurt that you did not tell me this before."

"I have tried, Frederika, but you have not been open to this conversation."

I said, "So, if Frederika were open to this conversation now, what would you want to tell her?"

"I have interests that are different than yours. I want to explore things, that have nothing to do with our marriage, but this does not mean that I don't love you. I want to be in a submissive relationship with a woman who can dominate me. I don't want that to be you. I don't think that would be good for our marriage, in fact, I know it would not. I cannot imagine you doing these things to me. I think it would be a turnoff to you and you might lose your attraction for me."

I said to them, "When you are sharing what you want, it is good to be specific about desires and avoid assumptions. Let's begin with how you are each feeling right in this moment?"

Pierre said, "I feel nervous and afraid that you will leave me now."

Frederika said, "I feel like I am not enough."

Pierre said, "No, that is not it. I want to try some things, maybe with a woman who will tie me up, maybe things that I know you don't want." "Does it make sense that Pierre wants something different?" I asked.

DIFFERENTIATED MONOGAMY

Being differentiated means that you each have different interests and are not merged into one person just because you are a married couple. Being a couple does not make you one person. This may be against popular current opinion, as our romantic version of love seems to be some kind of idealization of oneness, of completing the other, of finding one's other half. Love seems to be a perpetual pursuit of the other in order to complete an empty sense of self, one that is destined for emptiness and aloneness without a partner.

Through fairy tales and stories, our society teaches young girls about women who need to be woken up, who are asleep until a man comes along to wake them. These presexual women have no experience with life and remain in a dormant state until they are introduced to love through a more experienced adult male who is often times older and worldlier. With a kiss and the promise of marriage, he brings them to life.

Therefore, love in our society is attributed to longing, the waiting for completion, for the other to make one whole. Particularly for women, the lesson is that they should wait for the right man to come along, the one, the only, the perfect partner, the soul mate. This idealized partner will make them feel complete and they will never want for more or for another. Riding off into the sunset is the equivalent of the end of the road for a woman; she is complete, has finally found "the one," is on the road to marriage, and is never expected to want more. The fact that the fairy tales never show what happens after sunset, after dark, in the marital bed or the next morning, is a mystery to be solved over time in a desert of information. The lack of good sex education in this country leaves young people with the assumption that good sex comes only after an abstinent state of waiting, and that without explanation or education, magically appears in a lawful marriage with another often-inexperienced partner.

The *American Heritage Dictionary of the English Language* definition of differentiate is "To perceive or show the difference in or between;

discriminate and to make different by altering or modification, to become distinct or specialized; acquire a different character, to make distinctions; discriminate."[2]

Differentiate is an action word. It means to discriminate; to discriminate between two different things. When you differentiate you and your partner, you are discriminating between being two different people. As differentiated people you want different things because you experience different lives, even if you are together and are in the same marriage.

To be partners and yet be distinct from one another—to be differentiated—means to take on your own character and remain true to yourself. It means you can change from one thing and become something different. You can grow. Within a relationship there is a tendency to grow more alike as you age. But you don't have to become one person in two separate bodies. *Differentiated monogamy* means you take the action needed to mature as individuals. This may mean taking on a distinctive character as you age, growing into each phase of life, expanding and enhancing, emerging and maturing. You become distinct from your partner. This does not mean that you are not attached or connected. In fact, being in a differentiated relationship allows you to become more of who you are. You may both be in the same relationship, but the way you love each other gives you the permission you need to grow into separate people. This can help each of you discover more of yourself.

TIME, ATTENTION, AFFECTION, SEX

Relationships take four things to make them work: time, attention, affection, and sex. These four areas are the resources needed for your intimate life.

The experience of each of these things and their abundance will determine how connected you feel and how successful you think the relationship is. It will also determine how much you resent an outside relationship and give you important information on how to judge what is bothering you about what you're not getting or what you are afraid another partner is getting that you are not.

Gail and Gene, from chapter 3, opened their monogamy after Gene admitted he was having an affair with Dawn. His exploration had slowed down, but Gail's had increased dramatically.

Gene had finished a large painting and was about to head to his gallery for a show. Gail had been pasting flower petals onto a collage she was working on in her studio.

I asked them what, in the beginning, bothered them about their relationship. "Out of these four areas: time, attention, affection, and sex, which is the one that you need the most in your relationship, or what bothers you most when you're not getting it?" I asked.

"I need attention," Gene said. "It feels like she puts a lot of energy into giving attention to other people, and that bothers me."

"Well, Gene," Gail said, "we have been married for thirty-six years, how much attention do you need?" She laughed.

"See, this is what I mean. Of course she is going to pay attention to new guys. How could she not? How do I compete with all that new relationship energy? I get a little jealous of that energy."

New Relationship Energy (NRE)

One of the benefits of an open relationship is that it can keep the *new relationship energy* (what some people call *NRE*) flowing. It's possible to bring NRE into the marriage and keep the original love alive. Talking and communicating helps.

"For me," Gail said, "these relationships last a while. They aren't just one-night stands. But if I'm going to invest that time, the sex has to be different, some kind of kink or something different than what Gene and I have. I try to think about whether or not this works for me. Each person brings out a different part of me. I can be a different part of myself with each one."

As with Gail and Gene, all intimate relationships need attention. Intimate attention falls into these four categories: time, attention, affection, and sex. Where are you putting the most emotional labor in your current relationships? Do you focus on the time you spend together, sacrificing things you would rather be doing or people you would rather be with? Do you like self-care and dinner with friends, or do you pay attention to your kids and hobbies that you enjoy? Spending time with partners is crucial to making relationships work, but some relationships and some partners need more time than others. You might miss the affection in your primary relationship and turn to an outside or external relationship to compensate for the affection that's missing at home. Or you might miss the nonsexual physical touch between you and your partner and resent the touch they give their new, outside partner.

How do you feel about your sex life?

Imagine time, attention, affection, and sex as a pie with four slices. You may divide your pie slices differently than your partner. These four areas are all important, but one may be more labor intensive for you. You may enjoy one area more than another. What area do you want more of? Which makes you feel more loved?

Take a moment to think about each of these areas and make some notes about what you need and expect in each of your relationships.

What are your needs and expectations in each of these categories?

Time:

Attention:

Affection:

Sex:

Write down your thoughts and if you can, draw them out in a round pie shape. Make each slice of the pie equivalent to your needs in each area. You may have different pies for different partners. Or you can make a pie for what you are getting from your partner and one for what you actually want. It's easy to see from a visual perspective what you need. If you're ready, share your drawing with your partner or partners. Have a conversation about what each section, or slice, means to you. Most likely, they have a different definition for each area than you do.

Love is not a pie; you don't have less of one slice because someone else gets a bigger piece. But it can be helpful to see what you feel is missing or what you want more of. Remember, the more you love, the more there is to go around.

It may feel like there is a limited amount of time, attention, affection, and sex, but after further conversation you may find that there is an expansiveness to your relationship, a more open flow of give and take.

The "pie" analogy is simply a way to have a conversation about what you need in a relationship. Remember, love is not pie. But if you could have your pie and eat it too, would you feel like you had enough of what you wanted?

Things to Think About

Time: How much time do I need with my partner a week, and how much am I willing to let go of, so that they can be with other people? Am I comfortable with them having one night out a week? Overnight? A week night or a weekend night? What time of evening do they go out, after dinner or before? When do they come home, after I am asleep or do I wait up for them? If they come home in the morning, do they come home before I wake up or after breakfast?

Attention: What kind of attention do I need from my partner? Do I want to talk together without phones or other devices, particularly at meals, where we can share our thoughts and ideas? Is it important to me that my partner ask me about my day, or we connect at the end of the night by checking in about our feelings or experiences?

Affection: Is touch one of my love languages? If I were to express what type of affection I need from my partner, would it include the casual touch of their hand on my shoulder or arm, hugs, caresses, snuggling, or other forms of affection? Can I be very clear about what I need from them by showing affection in the way that I like it shown to me?

Sex: In thinking about the kind of sex that I want with my partner, can I open the conversation to include my own needs and desires? Can I have a frank and vulnerable talk about what would be problematic for me if they were to have sex with other people? What kind of sex is okay? What sexual behavior do we need to negotiate?

When you discuss these areas with your partner, decide how your areas differ and how they're alike. It is a good exercise to help you both realize what makes you feel intimate and connected, and how to spread those needs out over several relationships. As you try to balance your open monogamy, you will find that these terms come in handy.

Do you feel that your partner is spending too much time with someone else? Or are you just needing more affection when you are together? What are your needs and your expectations when it comes to sharing your partner with someone else?

We will discuss jealousy in a later chapter and how to deal with it. For now, this is a good place to start digging in to your more complex emotions and having direct conversations about how to balance your new life.

ට

CHAPTER SIX

A Promise You Can Keep

A good marriage is not determined by its participants but by its promise, and how well the partners can stick to it. To make a marriage work, it takes tremendous amounts of trust that the vow made at the time of the marriage is actually a promise that can be kept. If the promise can be flexible and fluid as the partners change, as their lifestyles change, as they grow developmentally, and as illness, parenting, finances, and life happens; if the promise and its meaning and the specifics of the problem can change, then the promise becomes a living breathing thing. *The promise is alive and grows with the couple.*

If, however, the promise is static, if it remains a one-time agreement in ancient language that has no meaning to the couple—because those words are quaint and traditional or because they bring comfort to your family and friends—over time, one or both partners will realize that the promise has no basis in reality for the way they are living and does not apply to them.

What makes today's marriage different is the commitment to a promise that can change, that can grow, that can be scrutinized for truths that apply to the moment and the space where the couple finds themselves today. In order to make a promise you can keep, you need to understand your own expectations and boundaries.

EXPECTATIONS

Most of us still place tremendous emphasis on the idea of monogamy. It feels like a guarantee of togetherness and exclusivity; it makes us feel that we are unique to each other in our love. Our promise says there is no one else who can usurp our place in the world, and this protects us from the threat of outside competition.

When you have an open monogamy, there are expectations as well. I call them *little m expectations* and *big M expectations*, as in little and big monogamy. Some expectations are less important to you than others, and some are crucial to your happiness and need more time for discussion. Your expectations can vary. They can be shared or your partner may disagree. It's important to keep the focus on the relationship, not on your expectation of your partner.

LITTLE M EXPECTATIONS

Some expectations may feel less important to your agreement. You may have less of an investment in the outcome, positive or negative. These smaller expectations around your relationship may mean less to you because there are smaller consequences if they are not met. You may not feel let down by your partner of they don't agree with your expectations or don't adhere to the agreement around these expectations.

For instance, Pat and Jane had been together for twenty years. They had defined their relationship as monogamous for eighteen of those years. They were a lesbian couple with a grown adopted daughter who was out of the house. Pat was fifteen years younger than Jane and was having a hard time letting go of their sex life. Jane was less invested in things staying hot and erotic. They liked to salsa dance and had been going to a club for years. Jane had no interest in continuing but was fine with Pat going to the club. Jane had a little m expectation that they would continue to dance and was not worried about Pat dancing with other women.

In my office, they sat at opposite ends of the couch. Jane pulled her sweater around her and Pat brushed her hair behind her ears. Jane was from Jamaica and had dark hair, with gray streaks. Pat was from the Dominican Republic and was small and curvy. She pulled her knees up and hugged them tight.

"This is not a big M expectation for me," Jane said. "There are more important things in our relationship."

I asked Jane if she could say more about her hopes and the possibilities for their openly monogamous relationship. It was new for them both and they were negotiating what was important. Talking about their big M and little m expectations was helping them to understand each other's viewpoints.

Pat said, "I have no hard and fast rule here. I want to go out and I want to dance. I am sad you don't want to go with me, but I am happy you are fine with me going. I want to know your rules or expectations for me when I am out; you know I love to flirt and dance all sexy."

I asked Jane, "What are the small or large things that you can live with and what are the things that you cannot live with? What will bother you?"

Jane said, "I have a hard line about you sleeping with someone and not telling me. Other than that, go out and dance, flirt, be sexy, make out with someone in the bathroom, all that is fine. Those times for me are over, I am sorry. But I know you want to do it. Have fun."

Pat said, "Okay, but what if I meet someone else? Someone new? You are okay with this?"

Jane looked at me for help. I said, "Every relationship is different. You can make up your own rules and expectations. Everyone has their own little m and big M expectations, and you should think about what's important to you."

BIG M EXPECTATIONS

In Jane and Pat's relationship, the big M monogamy expectations include how they each define their relationship. Jane considered her partnership with Pat to be primary. Any other partners they took on would have to be secondary or outside of their primary relationship. This was important to her. It was a big M expectation that she had for both of them.

She said, "Patricia, I do not want you to have another girlfriend. That is my big M, that is most important to me. You are my wife. You are the most significant person in my life. If someone were to replace me, I would be devastated."

Jane worried that if Pat felt differently, their primary partnership would be in trouble and she was not sure she could agree to the open relationship. She would have to revert to a more traditional monogamy agreement, where the two of them could only be with each other with no outside partners, no making out, no dancing, nothing. "This is my one big M expectation, I know it's crazy to think you would accept this, but, please?"

For now, Pat agreed. "I won't get into another relationship right now. I hear what you are saying."

I said, "Can this conversation be open for discussion in the future, if either of you meet someone you might want to bring into your relationship? This way, if you are both open to it, you can trust that the conversation will be brought up if the issue comes up."

Jane said, "Yes, I hope you will come talk to me if that happens."

"I understand that this is your big M expectation, Jane. I would not let you down," Pat said.

I said, "For Jane, this is really a redline, a very important boundary, and we should talk more about what this means."

REDLINES

When you consider your own big M expectations, they may include *redlines*, your hard boundaries. These are the personal lines that you would not step over, the boundaries that you have set for yourself and your own behavior. They may also be requirements you request of another person. You may ask that they respect your redlines and honor your boundaries. Your redlines are the places that you will not cross in order to protect yourself emotionally, physically, or psychologically. They are your own self-imposed limits, for your own good.

Some examples of redlines might be that you never lie to your partner, you never share details unless they ask, you don't sleep over at a new partner's house, you don't have intercourse without your partner being present, or you don't have sex with mutual friends. You may set these redlines as big M issues with your partner. They may be hard and fast boundaries that you feel you cannot compromise around because they have deep meaning to you.

I asked Jane, "It sounds like you are fine if Pat goes out salsa dancing and dances with other women, and even makes out with someone or has sex with them, but if I am hearing you correctly, you have a big

M expectation, an expectation of your monogamy agreement that she should not get into a serious emotional relationship with someone else. Is that a redline boundary for you? And if she crosses this redline, it is a real violation for you?"

Jane said, "I know that one of my redlines includes Pat being totally honest with me about making phone calls or connecting with people she meets outside of the salsa club."

"Wait, can that be a redline?" Pat asked.

"Redlines keep us safe," I said. "Jane feels like phone calls outside of the dance club are a hardline boundary for her. Does that make sense to you?"

"I guess," Pat said, sounding reluctant.

"Do you have any redlines for yourself, for the relationship agreement, or for Jane?"

"I do. My redlines include never sleeping over at another person's house unless we are together. I mean, if you go home to Jamaica, or I go to the Dominican Republic, that's different, but sleepovers are too personal, so, yeah, it's a hard no."

"So, Jane," I said, "are you hearing Pat that this redline is also a big M expectation, that she doesn't want either of you to have sleepovers with other people unless you are traveling home to Jamaica or the DR?"

Jane nodded.

I asked, "But tell me, Pat, does that mean if each of you are traveling separately, that you can sleep over with other people? I just want to make sure I get this right."

"Well, this brings up an interesting point," Pat said. "You know, Jane, that our friend is coming in from the city to stay at the yoga center. I want to visit them. Does that count as an overnight?"

Jane said, "Wait, this is your redline, Pat. You are already breaking it."

REQUESTS

A request is an "ask," something you put out to your partner hoping that they will agree. A request is not as important as a redline. A redline is about integrity; it is connected to your own personal belief system and stems from a certain set of behaviors that you operate from to stay true to the promises you make to your partner and to your agreement.

A request may be part of a smaller m expectation. Your partner can agree to it or not, or it could open further conversation.

In response to Jane's reaction to her interest in staying over with a friend, Pat said, "I am not interested in having sex with this person."

Jane thought about it for some time. "So, is this a request to stay with her, overnight, at the yoga retreat?"

I encouraged them both to think about the difference between their redlines and their requests. "When you think about the vision of what you want in your relationship, what do you imagine it would look like? Do you want freedom and openness to do what you each want, when you want? Or is the vision that you check in with each other before anything happens? Do you want to talk about things before anything progresses? How do you imagine this working?"

Jane said, "I've been thinking about this. I am fine with you going to see this woman. I know you are friends. But I know you are attracted to her. So, to be honest, I am fine if something sexual were to happen. I would *request* that for now, since this is new, you be cautious, and maybe just make out with her, for now."

"Okay, my request is that you trust me that this is all I will do," said Pat.

Jane said, "My redline is the same as yours. We should not be spending the night with other people. At least not yet. Spending the night with someone is a very intimate thing and I would not do that knowing that it would make you uncomfortable."

Pat looked at her and said, "I understand. This is a redline for both of us. No sleepovers. And that this is a big M expectation. I get it."

REFRAMING REQUESTS AS PERSONAL BOUNDARIES

I said to both Jane and Pat, "Can you frame your requests as personal boundaries, keeping the focus on your own behaviors instead of requesting things from your partner?"

"What would that sound like?" Jane asked.

"Try this," I said. "My request for my partner is _____ because my personal boundary is _____."

"Okay," Pat said. "I'll try. My request for you, Jane, is that you let me tell you what I did when I come home from dancing. Sometimes you don't want to talk about it, and it's important for me to bring that energy home to us. My personal boundary is that I can only do this if I talk to you about it. So, if you don't let me talk to you, it's like I can't get anything out of it and feel good about my own boundaries. Will you help me?"

Jane said, "I hear you. My request is that we wait until the morning to talk about your dancing escapades. My personal boundary is that I need sleep. Is that okay?"

They both laughed.

EMPATHY FOR YOUR PARTNER'S REDLINES

It is important, even if you don't agree, to empathize with your partner's redlines. If your partner is laying down a redline, it means that it is extremely personal and has meaning. Their redline is something that makes them feel safe, and when it is crossed, they feel like their agreement has been violated. Honoring it means listening openly and empathizing.

I said to Pat, "Let's go back and see if you can empathize with Jane's redline. You don't have to agree or feel the same, but you do have to try to empathize. Empathy would sound like, 'It makes sense to me, Jane, that your redline is no sleepovers. I understand that for you, spending the night with someone is a very intimate act and that you don't mind fooling around, or even having sex with someone else, but sleeping together for you has always been a true form of closeness and it's very special between you and me. It makes sense you don't want to share that with anyone else. Did I get that?'"

By empathizing, you are not agreeing, nor are you negotiating, nor are you promising to share the same redline as your partner. But empathy lets your partner know that you hear them, you get it, and you respect their right to have it.

Pat said, "It makes sense that you have this redline; it may mean that you are trying to make our open relationship work."

"It's in the big M column," Jane said.

As their relationship evolved over time, their redlines and requests changed. The more they communicated, they said, the less restrictions were placed on one another's behavior. They were able to find a freedom in allowing each other to try new things, with new people, if there was discussion about what was happening. Talking about feelings and consequences almost every day had at first seemed onerous and heavy. Now, they realized it made things easier, lighter. They had more freedom and fewer rules.

At home, Pat and Jane had an ongoing list on their refrigerator of big M and little m expectations. It was an ongoing "art" project, they said, with two columns, one with a big M and one with a little m and they each added things to the columns when they thought of new expectations. They also crossed things off when their requirements changed.

In the next session, I asked Jane if she had any other redlines or big M expectations, things that were important to their monogamy agreement. She said no, but Jane said she had a request.

"My *request* to Pat is that if she does go to see this friend, she calls me during the day. I want her to check in with me while she is with this friend so I know what's happening, what they are doing, and feel a part of it. I want her friend to know that I am here and that Pat is in a relationship with me, and that it's fine that they are together, that this is 'allowed' in our relationship. I want her to know that Pat is not sneaking around. Pat and I have an open agreement and I want this friend to know that."

HOW TO TALK ABOUT REDLINES

Whenever you talk about your redlines or requests, empathy is the first step. Once you feel you have empathized with your partner, it's important to next talk about your own feelings, and then for both of you to discuss the consequences of any actions. Like Jane and Pat, going through this process will help you and your partner have conversations about boundaries.

Jane's request for Pat to call her made sense to Pat. "Yes, I get that you want me to call you and now that you explained why, I understand that you want my friend to know that you are totally on board if anything happens. You want her to hear your voice, our voices together, so she knows we are a couple and we come first."

"Yes, I am not jealous, but maybe a little possessive," Jane said.

Pat replied, "That makes sense. So, let me tell you my feelings when I hear that. I don't mind you being possessive, in fact, it makes it kind of hot for me. I like that you want to be there with us, with her and me, and that we could somehow do this together, but not be in the same room. It's like I am taking you with me, but you don't have to be there so I can kind of do it myself. I like feeling like I have permission and a green light, and at the same time I am doing something that is outside of our old traditional monogamy like we had when we first got married. I feel excited."

Jane said, "I feel a little turned on as well. It's exciting and I feel morally we are doing the right thing because we are talking about it, we agree, we don't have to sneak around. I am still not sure if you are agreeing to my redline, although I hear that you empathize with me so I know you understand why it's important to me. If you know that it's important to me then I think you'll be more likely to respect my feelings about the overnight."

Pat said, "I will, and I feel the same, by the way, even though that's not always true with us and our redlines."

Now that Jane and Pat had talked about their feelings, I asked them to discuss the consequences. Consequences are the potential things that could happen, given their redlines and requests. Talking about consequences is a way to communicate specifically about what each of them imagines might happen. Our imaginations can create a beautiful vision of the future, or they can run away with a narrative that can lead to anxiety or even panic.

When discussing you and your partner's expectations, it's important to talk about the narrative you each have about what these wishes mean, or the meaning you assign to them. These potential consequences are the "stories" you make up about behaviors that haven't happened yet and what you imagine could be the result of those behaviors.

It's one thing to talk about your redlines, with their specific requirements in order to feel safe, and your requests, with their desire for promises from your partner, and yet it's another thing to talk about consequences. We each make up a story about what could or couldn't happen, about what our partner will or won't do, about things that we try to create.

You can both experience the same thing, on the same date, and it's likely it will be experienced differently. It will mean something entirely distinctive to each of you.

Sharing potential consequences means talking about fears, what you imagine might happen, the thoughts—both positive and negative—and how to handle your anxiety.

Sharing Redlines as Stories

This is an exercise that can help you talk about your fears over potential consequences if a redline is crossed. Share the narrative that comes up when you think about what your partner might do or is asking of you.

Share your reactions. What story do you make up?

When your partner shares a redline or a request, what does it bring up for you?

If I honor your redline:

If I don't honor your redline:

If I honor your request:

If I don't honor your request:

If you honor my redline:

If you don't honor my redline:

If you honor my request:

If you don't honor my request:

What I make up this means about you:

What I make up this means about me:

What I make up this means about us:

↻

For Jane and Pat, the conversation was focused on the consequences of what could happen if Pat went to see her friend. Jane said she thought some of the consequences might be that Pat would push to sleep over with her friend even though sleepovers were a redline for them both.

Pat looked at her with surprise. "I wouldn't do that."

"This is what I make up, Pat, not what is going to happen," Jane said.

I asked Jane to share what she was making up using the narrative sentences above.

"What does this mean about what you might experience or feel," I asked. "What do you make up?"

She said, "The story I make up is that I will be waiting all day to hear from Pat and maybe she won't call. She could forget about my needs because I am just not that important to her."

I asked Jane to describe the narrative she had in her head about what that meant about Pat, even though it might not be true. I told her to keep in mind that the story we make up is not really about the other person, it's about us, our experiences, and the lens through which we judge other people and our lives. It is often based on our past, our childhood, and what we have learned about life.

She said, "What I make up about Pat is that she really wants to be with someone else more than me. And she could push the edge of our agreement and pretend she forgot about it. She always does that. If I tell her to call me at five o'clock to let me know if she is coming home for dinner, she will work late and forget to call. She'll do the same thing with this. She will forget to call me and then tell me I should lighten up."

Pat said, "I would never tell you to lighten up. You are totally making that up."

"That's the point, Pat," I said. "We are exploring the narrative that Jane is making up. She is sharing her fears and the story that is running around in her head. It is not necessarily her truth or what she even believes; in this case it may just be her anxiety."

"Yes," said Jane.

"We will get back to this theme of feeling blamed or gaslighted, but before we do that, Jane, can you share the story you might be making up about what this means about your relationship?"

"What I make up about our relationship is that yes, I am anxious, but we are actually pretty solid, we are doing fine, we just need to talk about these things. I know we can talk about anything, the two of us, so we will be fine," said Jane.

They both looked at each other and Pat seemed to breathe a sigh of relief.

I asked Pat to share her stories, the ones she was making up about the potential date and how Jane felt about it.

"The story I make up about what this means about me is that our redline about not sleeping over is my redline too, so even though I am pushing boundaries and taking some chances, the story I make up is that I am growing into a more expanded person."

Pat continued, "The story I make up about what this means about Jane is that she is trying hard and being quite reasonable. And in our relationship, it means we can work through pretty much anything. I agree with her. We are doing pretty well with this."

By expressing their own stories instead of focusing on what was wrong with their partner, Pat and Jane could own their fears and insecurities and be heard by each other. It didn't matter if their stories made sense. What was essential was to get the conversation going by talking about what they each struggled with in order to talk about their feelings and concerns.

PRE-VENTING: HOW TO TALK ABOUT PROBLEMS

Pre-venting is a way to talk about potential problems before they become problems. Being proactive about potential issues before they become problems can prevent arguments and even breakups.

Most couples don't talk about their frustrations until they turn into resentments. Pre-venting can take a fear or concern and nip it in the bud. It is a way of talking about things in a proactive and transparent way in order to avoid problems later on.

I asked Pat and Jane to go back to the point that Jane had brought up earlier, about Pat's behaviors in the past and her frustration around Pat not calling and then blaming Jane for being too controlling.

"Can we pre-vent any possible problems that might arise here?" I asked. "If Pat does honor your request to call you during her time with her friend, that sounds like it will help a lot. If, however, she doesn't call, for whatever reason, it sounds like the story you make up is that she will act like it was too restrictive and then accuse you of being too limiting with your requests. Is that true? If so, can we pre-vent by discussing what might happen and how to prevent it?"

Jane said, "Yes, we can pre-vent this by having Pat agree to call me and then she can actually call me."

"Pre-venting is really talking about your feelings about something that hasn't happened yet. So, let's not make up that she won't honor your request," I said. "How can we talk about both of your feelings without blaming or shaming, especially for something that hasn't taken place and may not?"

Jane said, "I would feel hurt if Pat didn't call me. I would make up that she didn't care about me and I would probably be home making up all kinds of stories about what they were doing, and more likely, what they were saying about me. I would wonder what her friend thought of our relationship and of me and I would probably stay up all night waiting for her to come home so I could confront her."

"And if she did call you, as you asked?"

"Then I would, I think, feel relieved and I might be a little curious about what was happening, it could be exciting to think about. I wouldn't be jealous at all, it's just a sort of feeling of being on the outside but knowing I am totally on the inside, no one can replace me in Pat's eyes."

I asked Pat to empathize with Jane and then to pre-vent some of her concerns as well.

"I can see how Jane might feel anxious or upset if I didn't call her. But I can't see how that would happen, I mean I could make up a story where I might forget, but I would never do it on purpose. But after hearing how it would upset her, it's more likely it would be on my mind and I wouldn't be able to relax without calling her first. So, I imagine that I'd have to call her. My frustration, I imagine, is that I might feel trapped in that request. What would be a good time? How will my friend feel? Will it be awkward? Will it feel like I have to check in with my mother?"

Jane said, "Oh, well I don't want you to feel like I'm being your mother. I only want this to be fun for both of us. I can see how . . ."

Pat said, "I'm just making that up, right, we are talking about narratives here, things we are making up. I don't know if that's how I would feel, but it could be one reason why I wouldn't call. Not because I don't want to include you, I do."

"So, in order to prevent any hurt feelings or feelings of being parented here, what is a good way to resolve this for both of you?" I asked.

Pat said, "Well, I will call, but maybe we should have a time range that works for both of us. Maybe between four and five o'clock in the evening, so that you will know when to expect the call and I will know that I have to call and she will know I am calling."

"Yes, but even in your language you are saying 'I have to call.'"

"Okay, well I do, don't I?"

"No, this is not a redline for me, it's a request," said Jane.

"Okay, well I want to call. So, in order to prevent any bad feelings, I am telling you I want to plan the time. Does that work for you?"

"As long as you want to do it and you don't feel pressured. If you don't call, is it okay if I call you? I don't want to sit around and worry."

"Yes! Let's do that. That sounds like a good plan."

Pre-Venting

In order to pre-vent, discuss what might happen and how to prevent it:

If you/we _____ it's possible that
_____ (list any fears or concerns).

To prevent that, we could _____ (list ideas).

I would need _____
_____ (list things you can do).

I would appreciate _____
(list things your partner could do).

↻

Talking about potential problems and frustrations might seem like overkill to some. Some couples might need to work with a therapist or another third party to be able to handle the strong emotions and made-up stories that can overwhelm such conversations. But, like Jane and Pat, you can use pre-venting to help learn how to communicate and discuss the risks associated with letting other people into your relationship.

The success of your relationship is going to be determined by how open and transparent you are about your feelings—before, during, and after anything happens with any outside partners. This ongoing conversation helps release the bond of old narratives and sets you up to create a mutually agreeable open monogamy agreement.

CHAPTER SEVEN

Creating Your Open Monogamy Agreement

I f you are new to your relationship and just beginning the process of exploring the boundaries of your monogamy, then congratulations. You can start your relationship off in a healthy way by creating an open monogamy agreement. Going into a new commitment with these tools will allow you to create the relationship of your dreams. If you are rewriting your existing rules, good for you. If you are in total reboot mode, creating a new agreement between you can make all the difference.

In a phone interview from his home in Oregon, Leif recalled how he and his wife created their open monogamy agreement.

"Before my wife and I moved in together, many years before we were married, we made an agreement about nonmonogamy. And we reaffirmed and refined it before we got married. We wrote a complicated prenup, with two separate lawyers and the whole thing, which we then never needed to refer back to."

Some couples choose to craft an explicit legal document for their monogamy, with arrangements for property division and rules about shared custody. This can be done as a prenuptial or postnuptial agreement. Any requirements for open monogamy can be agreed to in writing using lawyers who are familiar with these types of arrangements and can help with the language. This is not necessary, but it can make some couples who have large assets or a history of betrayal feel more confident. For Leif, he realized that the legal document wasn't essential.

A prenuptial agreement that's signed and settled can provide emotional security and make both partners feel that the contractual obligation holds them accountable to the standards of the prearrangement. Yet, the spirit of a prenuptial agreement is that it holds you to financial repercussions in case of divorce. It is supposed to prevent one or both partners from taking advantage of the other. In this case, it may make the partners feel that their agreement is in writing and legally binding, but most attorneys will tell you that a contract cannot keep someone in a consensually nonmonogamous relationship, nor can it keep someone from cheating. It can, however, create consequences if one does break the agreement.

A legal agreement isn't necessary if both partners can create an open monogamy agreement verbally, or through writing, and trust the spirit of the agreement to hold each other accountable.

Accountability is different than liability. Liability is the state of being responsible for something by law. Accountability is the willingness to accept responsibility, to account for one's own actions, and maybe to even give reasons for it.

Discussing a monogamy agreement and what it might mean for both of you is important, whether you do it legally or verbally, through ongoing, continuous discussion.

Leif never needed to refer to his prenuptial legal agreement. After his wife passed away, he met Eugenia and didn't see the need to create a legally "binding" document.

"With my current sweetie, I had 'open' on my online dating profile before we even met. She still agreed to meet with me. We got along great, I really liked her right away. We discussed the idea of open monogamy on the second or third date."

Eugenia knew that Leif was open before she even went out with him, but she wasn't sure what that meant, exactly. They discussed the details during that date. He laid out his ideas of what it meant to be in an open relationship. He wanted some freedom to have other relationships, while at the same time being monogamous to the agreement that the two of them would make.

"I think for an agreement to work," Leif said, "it needs to really be agreed upon by all partners, not coerced. An agreement that seems unreasonable to one partner, that does not have real buy-in, is likely to be cheated upon. Which leads to lots of negative stuff."

Eugenia wasn't sure about it in the beginning, but she knew that Leif was special and that she came first in his life. They talked about it extensively and their agreement is clear. Underlying all their flexibility is the idea that they are primary to each other, and any other people they might want to have in their lives are secondary.

"Being clear on that and knowing that their partner is also clear on it is the key," Leif told me.

I asked Leif, "What are the most important things in your open monogamy agreement with Eugenia?"

He said, "Safe sex, flexibility, compassion, and care."

I asked him to say more about these things. They seemed like important boundaries for a monogamy agreement.

He said, "We have a safe sex agreement, which we both take seriously. We have discussed in detail what activities and what level of knowledge of our partners constitutes safe sex. We are both committed to keeping this agreement. There is flexibility in that agreement. Our agreement is very firm about condoms for PIV intercourse, though, but it includes the possibility that we might renegotiate. For instance, if one of us had a serious partner whose integrity and other attachments we both trusted, we might, after discussion and testing, include them in our *fluid bonded agreement.*"

Fluid bonded agreement

Fluid bonding means choosing to have sex with someone without protection, knowing that you will share bodily fluids. A fluid bonded agreement means both partners agree that this is acceptable with one another, or the agreement may be about fluid bonding with an outside partner. This is an important agreement when it involves more than two people. If a primary couple is fluid bonded, and they include an outside partner to be fluid bonded with, they are choosing to have unprotected sex between the three of them. This is a form of trust and intimacy as it puts the outside partner and all their partners at risk for sexually transmitted infections (STIs) and sexually transmitted diseases (STDs). All partners should discuss what makes sense to the whole system in terms of sexual health and emotional intimacy.

For many traditional monogamous relationships, there is an assumption that the couple has a fluid bonded agreement if they don't use protection. If sex is assumed to be part of their relationship and if they are only having unprotected sex with one another, the discussion about sharing bodily fluids does not have to include outside people, unless there is a betrayal to the agreement. When there are more partners involved, the risks increase exponentially.

There can be different and distinct levels of fluid bonding. After the primary couple has been tested for STIs, the discussion about fluid bonding with others can begin prior to any unprotected exposure.

Many STIs can spread without obvious symptoms, and some people think they don't need to be tested if they only have sex with partners of the same sex or if they have had the same partner for a long time. It is still necessary to be tested for a full panel of STIs to be sure there are no conditions that could be spread with sexual contact.

Choosing a fluid bonded relationship is complicated. It doesn't prove you care about a partner or how much you trust them. It might, in fact, show you care more if you choose to use protection. This is a discussion that you can have with all your partners in an open and honest way.

There have even been problems in Leif and Eugenia's fluid bonded relationship. They deal with these issues and practice empathy. Leif said, "Our agreement includes compassion for each other. There was an incident of a broken condom one time, and we handled it gracefully, with testing, and without blame or anger. We were honest about it. Honesty comes from trust. If we had less trust in our relationship it would have been so tempting for her to just not mention the incident. We take care of each other."

I asked, "That sounds like it was a stressful time. How do you deal with the stress when things happen between you?"

Leif said, "We always try to remember that we each have good will and love for the other, even in those times when we are not in agreement."

Having shared values of compassion and good will can prevent disagreement when things go wrong, which they inevitably will, as they do in all relationships. When there is a monogamy agreement that is, at its foundation, created with love and honesty, there is a "true north" to return to when life gets messy. That true north is the understanding you each have around what it means to share a complex, multifaceted life. We will go into shared values in greater depth in chapter nine.

EXPLICIT MONOGAMY AGREEMENTS

All partners who define themselves as a couple (and even couples who have outside partners) inevitably come to some kind of agreement about their monogamy, whether it is fully realized or not yet expressed. Monogamy agreements are implicit and explicit commitments regarding your expectations of fidelity.

An *explicit monogamy agreement* is what's said or committed to out loud by both partners. It defines the relationship's overt "rules" or structure. For many, this may, on the surface, forbid outside sexual or romantic involvements and usually has a timeline that is often "until death" of one party or the death of the marriage itself.

An explicit monogamy agreement can be a marriage vow or a partnership agreement that generally assumes and sometimes articulates both a personal and legal oath to the other person. We do this in front of our families, our communities, our church, our synagogue, or our mosque. This is a tribal type of commitment that we pass on through family, culture, and lineage, using words that are customary and personal to our families and may be handed down through generations. The words have meaning and they ring true on many levels. They feel right. They feel true. But when they don't, we alter and adjust them. We change them as we grow.

For instance, very few couples include the traditional language of "obeying" in their wedding vows—"I promise to love honor and *obey . . .*"—even though that wording may have been common practice only fifty years ago in most Christian wedding ceremonies.

We generally take our explicit monogamy agreement as a valid verbal contract and we take it seriously, regardless of whether we end up breaking it or changing it at some point in our marriage. *We believe in it, even if we don't necessarily maintain it.*

In research exploring marital values, over 80 percent of Americans polled said they thought infidelity was morally wrong. Of those who admitted to cheating, a majority said they didn't like to think of themselves as the "cheating kind." Even when committing infidelity, most people don't like to think of themselves as the kind of people who would break their monogamy agreement.

Most of us take our promises seriously.

We like to stick to our explicit monogamy agreements or at least like to think that we do. We humans, for the most part, consider ourselves to be honest and transparent. Yet, we can justify being unfaithful while at the same time believing we are being true to our promises. Most likely, when we make an explicit agreement, we have in our minds implicit assumptions about what that means.

When we make an explicit vow to be monogamous, most people fully intend to keep it, even though many end up cheating.

IMPLICIT MONOGAMY AGREEMENTS

The *implicit* monogamy agreement is different than the spoken, explicit monogamy agreement in that it may never be discussed at all. Often based on cultural mores, religious beliefs (or lack thereof), traditional sex roles, family background, and personal moral values, the implicit monogamy agreement may never be openly visited.

Each partner may hold a different, even opposing, understanding of what they think their agreement means. They may believe they are being true to their explicit monogamy agreement, but in fact are each following a different set of guidelines. Each partner may be expecting the other to follow the same set of guidelines but never discuss it, assuming they're both on the same page. This is why the idea of monogamy seems simple, and yet today's expectations about what the commitment actually means for each partner may be quite far apart on the spectrum of monogamy.

For example, implicit monogamy agreements might include things like "Talking to people online isn't cheating," or "I'm a guy and men can't help themselves," or "Going to strip clubs doesn't count as cheating," or "If it's only oral sex it doesn't count."

Other implicit assumptions include, "I'll be faithful until you stop having sex with me or I get tired of you, then I'll cheat," or "I'll cheat before I get divorced," or "If I stop being attracted to you, I'll cheat," or "If someone comes onto me, I won't be able to resist it."

The list of implicit assumptions goes on. If you are honest with yourself, you most likely have thoughts that are related to your own assumptions about monogamy and what it means to you.

These expectations come from past experiences, family values, gender roles, and cultural expectations. Sometimes negative views of marriage, fears or prejudices toward long-term commitment, or feeling forced into marriage for whatever reason can create resistance to monogamy, and those feelings are never discussed out loud.

Internal fears and sexist or misogynistic beliefs sometimes don't come to the surface until a conflict in the relationship triggers them. Both partners may be shocked to learn that repressed, hidden viewpoints lead to contrasting assumptions about marriage and monogamy. If not expressed, these assumptions can create feelings of betrayal later. These hidden feelings mean both of you have a belief about a nonexistent contract. Your marriage is not what you think it is. You need to get clear about what each of you are committing to.

Most couples never talk about their assumptions until a problem happens. To avoid a crisis, make your implicit assumptions explicit. This will help you avoid communication problems, expectation, and eventual disappointment.

The implicit assumptions about monogamy are often what precipitate a marital crisis. If you are having trouble in your relationship, or having doubts that you chose the right partner, it may be that you have committed not to the wrong person, but to the wrong agreement. Agreements can be changed. Expressing your feelings and being honest about your fears can mean the beginning of a new, more meaningful bond.

> Maybe it's not that you have committed to the wrong person,
> but that you've committed to the wrong agreement.

If you are feeling disappointed about your relationship right now, know that you can rewrite your monogamy agreement. You can have a monogamy that works for both of you. All it takes is openness, empathy, and understanding.

It is time to reboot your monogamy.

THE MONOGAMY GAP

The monogamy gap, as we discussed earlier in the book, happens when one partner wants to be more traditionally monogamous than the other. One of you may long for a more open relationship where you get to sleep with other people. You may want to experiment and long for more alternative types of sex. But your partner may have less desire for sex than you. They may want to be intimate once a week, while you want sexual connection of some kind every day, and you want sex with more variety, possibly more partners. This gap can cause friction and *communication fatigue*.

Couples who talk continuously about opening their monogamy but find they are revisiting the same topics over and over and getting nowhere can feel fatigued and frustrated. They get resentful and may end up hiding or lying to their partner.

Others feel that the constant scrutiny of their proposed behavior takes the juice out of anything that could happen. Managing the anxiety of the less-open partner can be tiring. And trying to share feelings and emotions beforehand can be frustrating for some people who find that just doing it and talking afterward can be more satisfying. It can also feel like the less-open person is blocking the more-open person by continuously demanding process conversations and dialogues when both partners don't feel that its helping.

This can then stop any change or growth in the open monogamy, which may unconsciously be what the more anxious partner is trying to achieve.

The exercises in this chapter can help. You will be communicating with each other, but the structure can help alleviate some of the communication fatigue. There is a beginning, middle, and end to these dialogues and you can choose how much you communicate and what will be helpful.

It is time to define, in a concrete way, what it means to you to be in an open monogamous relationship. No one can define that for you. Here, you will create your new monogamy agreement according to you own terms. You can make it loose enough to encourage growth and exploration with boundaries that make it feel safe.

The trick is to establish and continually revisit the rules so that you are conforming to your own set of values and you feel safe, but there is enough flexibility and transparency to feel free at the same time. You need safety to feel attached and you need freedom to grow, both within and outside of your relationship.

Some couples renegotiate rules about monogamy either directly or subtly as they age and pass through different developmental stages of their lives and their marriage. These rules can change when they have children, when the children go off to school or leave home, during menopause, at retirement, or when the spouses' roles change—if a wife or husband takes up a new career once the kids are out of the nest, for example.

Making an explicit monogamy agreement is like renewing your vows only without following a standard predetermined text.

> A monogamy agreement should be
> renewed at least every five years.

This is an agreement that you should revisit over and over, perhaps once a month, once a year, or at the very least, every five years. Maybe you are a couple that will want to discuss this every weekend. What matters is that your monogamy will remain something you can talk about for the duration of your relationship.

There is no right or wrong way to use the following exercises. This process can work for anyone. Whether you want to have sex only with each other, or you want to open your relationship and try being with other people, these exercises can help you integrate both your implicit and explicit monogamy, eliminating the monogamy gap.

CREATE YOUR NEW MONOGAMY AGREEMENT

The monogamy agreement is divided into sections that fall on the monogamy continuum. Each section has five questions that can be used for discussion. You may find that you fall more on the closed end of the spectrum for open monogamy. You might want a more secure monogamy and have a lower tolerance for any kind of outside relationship, including emotional relationships. Others might find that they fall more on the more fluid end of the open monogamy continuum. They want a more independent or autonomous open monogamy where they can each make their own decisions and do their own thing, where they don't have to check in with each other about each move they make outside of their partnership, and they can explore sexual experiences on their own. Or you could be somewhere in the middle. You might want to be flexible, and do some spicy things with some variety, but you always want your partner with you and have no interest in operating as a separate entity. There is no wrong or bad decision or a good or right way to do it. This is not a moral scale and there is no judgment; it is purely a way to begin a conversation. It will give you the structure you need to talk about opening your monogamy without feeling like you are free falling without a net.

THE MONOGAMY CONTINUUM

We reviewed the monogamy continuum in a previous chapter, but let's talk about what each section on the spectrum means. Remember, there is a range, and you don't have to fit perfectly in any of these categories, you and your partner don't have to agree, nor is there a right way to operate within each category.

Closed

A closed monogamy agreement is a traditional, monogamous agreement where any and all sexual and emotional connection stays between the primary partners. There may not be any discussion of fantasies, and masturbation is kept private or is a secret. This category can be very repressive when partners feel they have sinned in their hearts if they lust after another, or it can be deep, soulful, meaningful, and intensely erotic. Even within a closed monogamy there is a spectrum.

Fantasy

The fantasy category of open monogamy is where a couple shares their fantasies openly, and those fantasies can include fantasies of other people. This may include watching pornography together, and whether they do it together or separately, it does not threaten the relationship. In this category it is not considered a breach to imagine being with someone else.

Some couples can share those thoughts with each other and use that erotic energy for their shared sexual pleasure.

Emotional

An emotionally open monogamous relationship means that emotional relationships and romantic flirtations may be acceptable, depending on the agreement. These types of relationships can be tricky. Without a conversation and an open agreement, an emotional relationship could either be a friendship or a full-blown emotional affair. Emotional affairs are hard to define and even more difficult to negotiate. The simple way to determine if you're having an emotional affair is this: if you are hiding and lying about a relationship, even if there is no sex or physical contact, it's probably an affair. Couples who can talk about their emotional connections with others will talk deeply about privacy, freedom, friendship, and trust.

Sexual

The sexually open monogamous relationship can mean many things, but in general, it is defined as being sexual with others when both partners are present. It may mean watching others have sex, or it could mean having sex with each other while other people have sex. It can also mean that you and your partner participate in sex parties together. There is a wide range of possibilities here, all of which can be discussed as the opportunities are created.

Autonomous

The autonomous category is sometimes an extension of a sexually open relationship. It means one or both partners can explore sexual and romantic connections, while keeping their primary partner as the top priority. People in these relationships tend to tell their partner everything, before and after, and sometimes during. There is never anything that happens that both partners are not privy to and everything is discussed at length, including jealousy or other concerns. These concerns are respected and take priority over the desire for outside stimulation.

Independent

Partners who are independent in an open monogamy can explore sex with other people and follow their own limits. They often pursue sexual and romantic desires, acting independently of their partner. They feel that no one should tell them how to live their life, including their sexual life. Their sexual behavior is private, and their partner feels better not knowing. These people appreciate their partner's capacity to grant them sexual freedom and limit the relationships outside their primary partnership, keeping their marriage central. Sometimes it is only one partner who is independent while the other partner remains monogamous.

Unlimited

In unlimited open monogamy agreements both partners are allowed unlimited sexual, emotional, and romantic relationships without having to report in to the other or having to ask for permission. They may have a don't ask, don't tell policy with one another. There is no need to share the experience afterward, unless they agree it would be beneficial to them both. They may use their outside experiences to bring erotic or romantic energy into the marriage, but they don't have to. It is understood that seeing other people does not mean they are on a path to divorce or breaking up. It works for both partners until it doesn't.

Poly

Polyamorous couples have physical, emotional, affectionate, romantic, bonded, and sexual relationships with other people, within their marriage. They can bring in other partners and may share households and child rearing duties either part time or full time. There are a number of distinct relationships within a poly group such as primaries, secondaries, and metamours. There tends to be more conversation and open dialogue between the original partners in poly relationships. The polyamorous often don't like to identify as monogamous at all. The term seems contraindicated and is offensive to some.

Relationship Anarchy

In relationship anarchy there are no hierarchical primary or secondary partners. All partners are treated equally and the original partners are not necessarily primary. The idea is that no societal structure can determine how they should love. The disruption of traditional stereotypes and gender roles says that anything goes here and rules of any kind about marriage or committed partnership is a form of control and a type of repression. Equity and inclusion are key.

Detached

Although one might wonder why detachment is part of the monogamy spectrum, it makes sense that when one or both partners pull away from the partnership they can reach a developmental phase of monogamy or end up on the far end of the monogamy continuum. By being disinterested or withdrawing from the relationship, the detached partner is holding the still-interested partner hostage to an agreement they are no longer upholding. When one partner no longer wants a sexual or intimate relationship but they don't want the other partner to go outside the relationship, that is just as much of a betrayal to their monogamy agreement as cheating might be. The implicit assumption of marriage or committed partnership, unless otherwise explicitly stated, is to have a sexual partner for life. When one partner stops or prohibits that, for reasons other than illness, the relationship suffers and the agreement is breached.

As you review these categories of monogamy you may find things you want to explore, or these definitions might make things more confusing for you. Maybe you don't need a definition for your relationship. Or maybe you are still exploring.

Try the exercise below. Going through the questions may give you clarity and allow you to think more clearly about what you want, at least for now.

This is not a quiz. There is no score at the end. It is only meant to open up areas of discussion in each category.

ANSWERS IN THE PRESENT

After you have discussed your answers to the questions below, you might want to write out some of the things you agree on. You'll find a sample at the end of the monogamy continuum exercise below. Or you can create your own.

Your commitments, or the things you agree on after talking about the issues below, should be worded in the present tense. Describe them as if they are happening now. For instance, "We are having sex once a week. We are open to trying new things. We will talk about it right away if one of us wants to have sex with someone else. We will discuss before, during, and after a date and process any feelings of jealousy."

Don't worry yet. Start by having the conversation. Answer the questions in the best way you can and discuss them together.

Finding Your Place on the Monogamy Continuum

The following questions are based on the categories of the monogamy continuum. Use them to open a shared discussion with your partner. Take your time and either write down the answers to the following questions first or discuss them in real-time with your partner.

This is an introduction to building your new open monogamy agreement:

Before You Begin:

Start with an appreciation for one another and end with an appreciation for one another. Appreciation is important, as it moves you into a place of receptivity and connection.

One thing I appreciate about you right now:

My intention for doing this exercise:

What I hope we get out of it:

Closed

What topics are important to talk about with each other?

What is private and what is secret?

How do we bring up subjects that might be awkward?

If we have resentments, should we share them or keep them to ourselves?

If we have thoughts about changing our agreement, should we bring them up?

Fantasy

If we have sexual fantasies, should we tell each other?

Is it cheating if we imagine being with someone else?

If we have fantasies, can we share them with a friend?

Do we watch pornography together?
How often? Who picks?

If we have fantasies we want to act
out, how do we bring them up?

Emotional

Does flirting count as cheating?

Can we talk to strangers on social media?

What constitutes an emotional affair?

Should our emails be transparent or private?

What things are private between us
and not okay to share?

Sexual

What if we want to have sex with someone else?

Can we have sex with someone else together?

Is watching other people have sex a
threat to our relationship?

Can we have sex with other people
when we are not together?

How do we start the conversation if we
want to expand our sex life?

Autonomous

What if one of us wants to do something
sexual, do we tell the other?

What if one of us gets turned off by
the other person's desires?

What if one of us desires a different type
of sex than we are currently having?

What if we are convinced that the other
person will not be into this type of sex?

What would be a safe way to talk
about things if we feel jealous?

Independent

Are we monogamish, and if so, what does that mean?

Do we pursue our own sexual desires no matter what?

Who is in charge of improving our sex life?

If one of us wants more sex than the other, does
that determine how often we have sex?

Can we have sex with other people
and not tell each other?

Unlimited

Should we talk about our dates with other people?

Can we tell other people about our unlimited dating?

Do we use our experiences outside the partnership
to turn us on when we are together?

Does unlimited mean the same thing
to me as it does to you?

If one of us wants to dial it back,
what is our agreement?

Poly

When do we have the conversation about opening
our fluid bonded agreement to others?

Do we have to give approval to let in a poly partner?

When do we introduce a poly partner
to our kids or extended family?

Is it possible a poly partner might
live with us someday?

What are the guidelines for dating and
spending time with others?

Relationship Anarchy

Are ex-lovers off limits?

How do we talk about transgressions?

How often do we spend time together?

How do we feel about sharing?

What if we feel like one of us is becoming
less important than others?

Detached

What if one of us doesn't feel aroused in
bed, should we have sex anyway?

What happens if we don't have sex for a
week or a month or several months?

If we become detached emotionally,
how do we talk about it?

Can we live together as companions and not be lovers?

If one of us wants to end our
relationship, do we fight for it?

Extra Questions

Add any other questions that you think are important. Some
examples may be:

How do we divide chores?

How do we divide child care?

How often do we see your parents? My
parents? Other family members?

Will we have sex after childbirth? How long after?

How often do we go for couples therapy?

Who initiates the therapy?

When do we retire?

Where do we live after we retire?

Now, add your own questions:

When You Are Done:

Take some time to process this exercise using the questions below. You may have done this all in one sitting (wow) or it could have taken you several days or even weeks to complete. This can be part of an ongoing discussion, one that can expand to include new questions and to discuss and explore new desires as they occur to you.

One thing I appreciate about you right now:

What I feel having done this exercise:

What I got out of it:

○

YOUR OPEN MONOGAMY AGREEMENT

Once you are satisfied with the answers to the questions above, you can write out your answers in the following open monogamy agreement format.

Some things you may agree on. Other answers may lead to more questions or even conflict. This is just a conversation starter. It does not have to be written in stone and no one has to agree on anything for now.

Be as clear as you can. Although your monogamy agreement might seem explicit, with a black-and-white edict, it may be more indefinite than you think. For example, "No having sex with other people" is vague. For some, this means no intercourse with anyone other than your spouse. For others it could mean no posting bathing suit photos of yourself on social media. In every relationship there are implicit assumptions. Monogamy is not one blanket set of rules; it has permutations, it has hard and soft limits. Your monogamy should be designed to fit you as a couple, to encompass your personal needs and your viewpoints.

It can be helpful to write down three categories, keeping in mind they are flexible and fluid and will be revisited often. For now, what are you questioning? What are you considering? What are you committing to?

In our open monogamy agreement,

We are questioning:

We are considering:

We are committing to:

Dated:

Signed:

We will renew this agreement on:

For instance, Pat and Jane added the following to their open monogamy agreement:

We are questioning:
Whether to visit an old friend together

We are considering:
Spending the night with her, as long as we are together

We are committing to:
Talking every week in therapy about this new agreement

FOLLOWING UP

Whether you make your agreement using this format or another, make it fun. Sign it and keep it somewhere safe. Remember, this is not a legal agreement. You are not liable, but you are accountable. Revisit the monogamy agreement anytime you are unsure about your commitment.

Decide when you will review the agreement. Make an appointment. Discuss how and when you want to update it. Let there be time for questions and then revise as needed. Remember, the questions you used for discussion are just an introduction to the topics you can discuss in your new open monogamy agreement. Make sure to add your own questions for discussion and revisit your agreement often.

Your new open monogamy agreement is one of the most important things you will accomplish in your lifetime. It should not be taken lightly or dismissed easily. Give yourselves credit for having created a conscious relationship and then congratulate yourselves for moving forward in your relationship. Now, take the time to celebrate. Have a ceremony or ritual that commemorates the experience for you.

WHY DO IT?

Having one partner to focus on and grow a deep and intimate connection can be wonderful. With one partner, you can soulfully expand into new and different experiences, which can lead to a rewarding and satisfying life.

If you are challenge averse and would rather avoid conflict and prefer to deal with one partner at a time, then conventional monogamy may be more than enough.

If you crave fulfillment with a variety of sexual partners and find personal growth and development with multiple people, an open monogamy might be for you. If you can tolerate perpetual exploration of emotions, are emotionally astute and insightful, and don't mind long hours of processing, you can probably handle an open relationship.

Other people say the reason they want a consensual open relationship is to experience greater amounts of love. Love is extensive and grows the more you share it. Love is not a pie; you don't divide up love. Your time, attention, sex, and affection might be limited, but people who want open monogamy say that the depth of their love for their primary partner increases when they have more choices. They are able to love multiple people and that gives them the ability to give love and experience even more love. The comparison has been made to having multiple children. If you're a parent, you know that having more than one child does not decrease your love for any of them. Your resources might be diminished, but love doesn't decline and you love each one in a different way.

Those who seek open relationships don't have to break up with one person to be with someone else. (Imagine having to give up one child in order to have another, one interviewee told me.) Open partners can have new love, without letting go of old love. There is no grading system and no one love which is greater than another. They feel they don't have to trade in one to have the other. They may feel more responsibility for a primary partner, but love is not about that.

Some may see having multiple partners as being selfish, the desire to "have their cake and eat it too." But really, what's the point of having cake if you can't eat it? That's a senseless expression. If anyone thought about it for more than a second, they'd realize we all want cake that we can actually eat, not just look at.

The feeling of falling in love is one of the greatest human experiences the body and mind will ever have. For those lucky enough to love at least once, there is no comparison. To love more than once is a gift. To love several people at the same time, well, it's like having cake, being able to eat it, *and* not being gluten intolerant. Or not gaining weight or getting cavities.

What if you could have your cake, eat it, have a different flavor whenever you wanted it, and nothing bad happened? What if you just lived your life and didn't hurt anyone? Open monogamy might mean you could just be happy. And you can love the cake. And it can love you back.

CHAPTER EIGHT

What If It Doesn't Work?

Ending an open monogamy agreement doesn't have to mean the end of your relationship. It can just mean you are starting over. If things don't go as planned, begin a new agreement. If what you have created doesn't work for you now, based on where you are in your relationship, you can create something else. You have choices. You can dial things back or open things up; you can be flexible.

You may not have been aware of it, but you have always had an implicit agreement. Now you know what it takes to make everything explicit. If what you agreed to is not working, you now know how to change the rules.

You may have made some mistakes along the way. You may have tried things that one of you didn't like. Hopefully you learned some things about yourself and have communicated in more open ways than ever before. It is the commitment to fluidity that is your new challenge. You know that there are endless choices and possibilities. When there are so many choices, you might feel pressure to make the right ones. Especially if things have gone off the rails.

Usually when something doesn't work it's because you tried something that doesn't line up with your values. The internal conflict kicks in and you realize this is not the relationship you thought you'd have.

Think about the moment you knew you were "ready" to commit to your partner, to a relationship, or maybe to marriage. Did you just know, or was it a process? How did you know that this one person, among the millions of options on the planet, was going to be your person? How did you choose? Did you decide that choosing them meant giving up alternative options? What was your internal conversation? Go back to that moment and see if you can find that turning point, that place where you made a choice, where you picked this particular person among all others. When you first met your beloved, what did you know in that moment?

Open monogamy is a process too. It takes time to find where you are comfortable and what feels right. You might have to push the edge and then shut things down. You might expand into scary places and then pull back. It might not happen all at once. You might not find the sweet spot, the place that feels safe for both of you, right away.

THE DESIRE DROP

When you first fell in love you probably felt really strong emotions, maybe even passion and an intense desire for your partner. And you have been trying to maintain those feelings ever since. Maybe they are still there, and you are still hooked. Maybe it still works, and your passion for each other will be everlasting.

For most couples, these feelings naturally change over time. When your desire wanes, it can feel like your love does as well. When the new relationship energy wears off, you may feel the drop, the loss of that intense desire, and wonder who or what to blame. You might blame yourself, or them, or you might wonder if it's monogamy in general. You thought you would love this person the same way you did when you first met. Intellectually, you may have recognized that things change, but you wanted to maintain the passion. When it wanes, it can feel like things are breaking down.

In the recent The Good Wife Study by the dating site Ashley Madison, 64 percent of women claim they are no longer attracted to their spouse at all and say a "physical change" in their partner is the primary catalyst for their online affair.[1] It's true that as we age, our physical appearance changes. Most likely, we grow tired of our partners and the desire decreases as the resentments and frustrations of long-term captivity settle over us. Seventy-four percent of women in the Ashley Madison study still love their spouse, but aren't turned on by them.

Of those same women surveyed, 64 percent said they felt sexually neglected in their marriage and 43 percent said their marriage is sexless. Sometimes people start outside relationships to stay married.

SHOULD MARRIAGE HAVE AN EXPIRATION DATE?

It makes sense in these days of high divorce rates, serial monogamy, and the decrease in sexual fidelity within marriage, to include an automatic re-up, a renewal, that's built into marriage. For instance, after five years a couple could meet and discuss the terms of their marital agreement to decide if the marriage should be terminated or renewed. Only when both partners agree to renew should the contract be continued. The new marriage contract would then be reviewed every five years by both partners and all the terms revised as needed. The contract would be written out in clear language, with the terms spelled out. The clauses would include things like the division of assets, parenting and childcare, and sexual possibilities, in detail, for the current round of renewal.

This could create a unique solution to the problem of high divorce rates. There would be no need for a huge wedding every five years, but there could be a renewal ceremony every cycle to celebrate the new contract.

If this became part of our regular expectation, would we appreciate our time together in a new way? Would we celebrate our renewals like anniversaries, but bigger and better? Or would these renewal ceremonies be smaller, more personal, but more meaningful? Would we learn to let go, end things, and say goodbye in a more mature, less painful way when our time together came to an end?

We are familiar with the act of making long and short-term commitments in our lives. We sign loan agreements, take on mortgages, and start new jobs. When we buy a new phone, we sign an initial contract, although buyers rarely, if ever, read what they are agreeing to. Think about your personal comfort level with commitments. Do you feel more content in shorter or longer commitments? What would give you more security, a two-year, a five-year, or the standard thirty-year mortgage? How does this relate to your marriage cycle? Or to the many stages within a committed relationship?

What is the life cycle of your average relationship? Some say that our lives naturally shift in seven-year cycles, just as the skin cells of our body rejuvenate every seven years and we have all new skin on our bodies, becoming essentially a new person. Would you rather have a relationship life cycle that coincided with your natural life experiences instead of a life sentence that committed you perennially to a partner? Our life cycles can coincide with a concerted effort to create an agreement that is based on feelings, and we can commit to the agreement knowing there is a beginning, middle, and end.

What is the value of your current experience and how would knowing that your relationship must be reevaluated affect how you treated your partner or your time together?

Questions to Ask:

What are my goals for the next five years?

What are our goals for our relationship for the next five years?

If the person I am in five years could give the person I am now a message, what would it be?

If the person I was five years ago could give me a message, what would they say?

CHEATING

Cheating is as old as mankind (or womankind). Nonmonogamy within marriage has been around forever. Nonconsensual nonmonogamy, or cheating, has been the flip side of marriage for thousands of years. Particularly common throughout history are men who have taken outside partners and women who have turned away or denied it was happening.

Adultery happens in every culture, all over the world. In Wednesday Martin's book *Untrue*, it states that research shows that women have had affairs as often as men; they have just been better at hiding it.[2] In some cases, there may have been advantages to having multiple partners, both sociologically and genetically. A woman could guarantee pregnancy if she had multiple sexual partners, thereby assuring the perpetuation of the species. That said, it is not biologically proven that men "spread their seed" to ensure reproduction. That theory is based on a 1940 experiment done on fruit flies that was never reproduced with animals or humans.[3] It is more likely and better researched that females are promiscuous in order to guarantee impregnation.

Helen Fisher, an anthropologist, agrees. She says women have always cheated at the same rate as men, but they have also had more motivation to hide their adultery, since there are more negative and many times more dangerous consequences for them when they are caught.[4]

In 2019, the dating site Ashley Madison found that there was one active female account on their site for every one active paid male account. They have had more than 5.6 million signups in the past year alone, with an average of 472,777 new signups per month and more than 15.5 thousand new accounts opened daily.[5]

Male or female, infidelity means not only breaking your monogamy agreement with your partner, but it may also betray the agreement you had with your own love story. This is why infidelity can feel traumatic not only to the person who is cheated on, but also to the person who cheats. The person who cheats is betraying their own sense of integrity and their belief in who they are as a person and as a partner.

Open Relationships and Cheating

An open relationship doesn't protect you from infidelity. Things are just more complicated. Not only are you breaking your commitment to be honest and transparent with your partner, but you are cheating on everyone else involved as well. It could be just your spouse and one other partner who is affected, or you could be betraying everyone in a many-layered, multi-tiered polyamorous pod. If you break the agreement you have with your spouse or with your poly-pod, you are cheating on all of them. It doesn't matter if you neglect to mention you went out for coffee with someone after promising to tell, or if you have a full-blown sexual and romantic parallel marriage on the side. If you make a promise regarding your emotional or sexual fidelity and you break it, it's a betrayal.

Affairs affect about one-third of all couples.[6] According to data collected by the *Journal of Marital and Family Therapy*, 57 percent of men and 54 percent of women report that they cheated.[7] Infidelity statistics are hard to measure with pinpoint accuracy because infidelity is based on dishonesty and people lie to the researchers. Men tend to brag about their affairs while women will minimize their infidelity. Many books and articles written about affairs assume infidelity is a symptom of fundamental problems within a marriage or committed partnership. This assumption of foundational problems is not true and it is victim blaming. It also ignores a more fundamental question: Is monogamy the exception rather than the norm?

Affairs Don't Solve Relationship Problems

Traditional monogamy may be an impossibly high standard for the average person. *This is not an excuse for you to justify your affair.* Just because monogamy is hard doesn't mean you can't do it. Many people, in fact two-thirds of people who enter relationships, are able to stay true to their partner.[8] They may not be happy in their marriages, but they don't cheat (or, at least they hide their cheating well).

It's rare for people to end up with the person they cheat with. Only 3 percent of people who have affairs marry the person they cheat with.[9] Maybe this is because a good majority of people who cheat are not doing it because they are unhappy or dissatisfied with their marriages. Studies show that up to 56 percent of men and 34 percent of women who have affairs described themselves as happily married. They also said they were having good sex and loved their primary partners, even at the time of the affair.[10]

What Is an Affair?

There are three parts to an affair. The first is that there is an outside relationship of some kind. It may be online, an emotional relationship, or a full-blown love affair. It could be a work spouse or a sex worker.

The second part of an affair is the sexual component. The sex can be over a webcam or masturbation to porn. It can be with someone of the same sex you are primarily attracted to or with someone of the opposite sex you tend to be attracted to. It can be with a sex worker, or it can be kinky sex where there is role-play but no genital contact.

The third part of an affair is the dishonesty. There can be voluntary disclosure and full confession, or unintentional discovery with denial or gaslighting, hiding, and cover-ups.

For most couples, the hardest part of an affair is the dishonesty. Preventing lying and hiding can be one of the motivators for opening a relationship. If you are honest about your outside relationships, then ostensibly, you don't have to hurt or betray your partner by lying about it. But if you have an open relationship agreement, lying about an additional relationship can be even more confusing and perhaps more devastating.

Outfidelity

Outfidelity is how I refer to an affair or betrayal in an open marriage. Usually, a partner reveals that they have been keeping a secret about one of their relationships or cheating with someone outside of their agreed-to partnerships.

If the open monogamy agreement includes transparency about all outside partnerships and the primary partner has agreed upon all potential dates, both romantic and sexual, everything is supposed to be out in the open. The couple can have relationships with other people as long as there is full honesty and transparency between the primary partners. When one partner acts outside of that agreement and keeps something a secret, it is a betrayal to the open agreement. And when they disclose the cheating to the partner, it's called outfidelity because the betrayal is to the primary partner as well as the whole system, which includes any secondary or tertiary partners.

Infidelity happens in a traditionally monogamous relationship when a partner cheats on another partner. Outfidelity happens when a nonmonogamous partner cheats on their open partners.

The spouse who hears the disclosure is expected to try to respond with an open mind and with empathy, to try to work with the cheating partner to understand what happened. This can be difficult, as difficult as any conversation about infidelity. The most important thing in an outfidelity conversation is to try to figure out why the partner thought they couldn't share sooner, and to determine the level of continued trust in the relationship.

Open Monogamy Is Not . . .

Sometimes people try to use an open marriage as an excuse to continue an affair. They will get caught cheating or confess and try to negotiate the continuation of the infidelity with permission. They may make the partner feel coerced or bullied, or like they have no other choice but to acquiesce to an open agreement. Continuing an affair is not part of an open marriage.

Elisabeth "Eli" Sheff, a researcher, author, and expert in polyamory, said, "Polyamory shouldn't be a Band-Aid for a failing monogamous relationship."[11]

It's up to both partners to create an agreement that makes them feel secure in the relationship that they share.

When Your Partner Has Had an Affair

Questions to ask the partner who cheated in an open marriage:

Why did you feel you needed to keep this outfidelity a secret?

Was this person you were with someone we had vetoed in the past?

Was it someone you assumed would be vetoed if you asked me about them?

Did you get an emotional or sexual charge by hiding this relationship?

Does your connection to this person violate one of your personal boundaries?

What details can you tell me about how this began and why it went underground?

What are you still wanting to keep secret or private about this relationship?

Are you willing to let go of this or do you want to continue the relationship?

What do we need to change in our agreement as a result of this?

When You Are the One Who Cheated

If you are the one who cheated, answer these same questions and be as honest as you can in your answers. Write out your thoughts first. Be clear about how you want to address things before you have the conversation. Thinking things through can help.

○

JEALOUSY

Many people assume that an open relationship will cause jealousy in both partners. Some argue that jealousy is a sign of healthy attachment, a feeling that proves love and connection. Historically, it has been assumed that pair-bonded individuals who are attached in a "healthy" way are sexually exclusive, and that exclusivity is an indicator of the success of their romantic pairing. Therefore, jealousy should be a hallmark of a successful relationship.

Instead, research has found that some pair-bonded partners experience positive feelings instead of jealousy when they open their relationship.[12] This means that a healthy bond is not necessarily threatened by opening things up. If you are secure in your relationship and know and trust your partner, that solid attachment may supersede the need for jealousy.

Jealousy is about fear. It's the fear that someone else might get more of your partner or take something that you already have. Jealousy feels like someone else will threaten your bond. And they might.

But feeling jealous doesn't mean there's something wrong with you. It's a normal emotion. Jealousy shouldn't be ignored. Sometimes it's a warning. It can be a canary in the coal mine, a way to identify problems in a relationship. It can be an indicator that there are threats from competing sources. It's important to listen to your intuition. Jealousy can be a sign that your partner could be straying from your relationship. Sometimes, it's an early warning system.

But some people don't experience any jealousy.[13] They find delight and pleasure in their partner's sexual experiences with other people or outside relationships. This does not necessarily indicate a problem. It may be a type of generosity. The ability to see your partner as a totally differentiated person who can appreciate other people is an expression of love. "Letting" your partner receive love from others without worrying that it will take something away from you is a sign that you are secure in your relationship, and in yourself. These people may experience *compersion* or pleasure in their partner's happiness with someone else.

Most people in open monogamy relationships aren't interested in leaving their primary partner for anyone else. They prefer being with each other and don't want to break up; they want to share their lives. But they also want to share other experiences and discover other parts of themselves with other people. That doesn't mean you won't ever feel jealous.

HOW TO DEAL WITH JEALOUSY IN AN OPEN MONOGAMY RELATIONSHIP

It can be hard to deal with jealousy.[14] The emotion can make you feel tense and can be emotionally or even physically painful. Jealousy is triggered when you think of your partner with someone else. It could be with a specific person or in a particular sexual situation. Jealousy can come and go, and can get stronger and more intense, depending on your partner's response to your emotions. If they get defensive or deny your feelings, it can make you more suspicious and increase your distrust.

There are many ways to deal with jealousy, but the first step is to focus on your own feelings. We will talk about how to deal with your partner's jealousy next.

First, confront the jealous feelings in yourself. Admitting you're jealous is hard, but discovering where the feelings are coming from can help. What are you afraid of? Are you concerned about the time your partner is spending with another person? Are you worried about the attention they are giving them? Or the affection, or the sex? Can you get specific about what is bothering you?

Next, talk about your fears. Ask your partner if you can sit down and have a real, honest discussion about your feelings. Be as definitive as you can about what it is—the time, attention, affection, or sex—that is making you jealous.

Statements to Start a Discussion:

I am feeling some jealous feelings.

When you ____ it makes me feel ____.

I might be doing ____ to participate in some of those feelings.

I need ____ from you right now.

Finally, take an honest look at your feelings. Investigate your layers of jealousy. Could there be other feelings underneath your jealousy? Is there curiosity or even interest when you think of your partner with someone else? Could you imagine changing your feelings of jealousy to compersion?

COMPERSION

Compersion is the feeling of happiness or satisfaction when you see your partner with someone else. In one study on jealousy and compersion, researchers found that a secondary partner could enter into a relationship without creating jealousy between the primary partners.[15] The primary partners often felt possessive of the other, but without feeling threatened or angry about their "other" relationship.

Susan Wenzel, author of *A Happy Life in an Open Relationship*, has a good guide for dealing with jealousy. I spoke with her as she was writing her book and dealing with her own open relationship issues. She came up with the following list of questions to ask yourself to help navigate jealous feelings:

How do you experience jealousy?

What are your thoughts and feelings about the situation that are causing this jealousy?

What story are you telling yourself? For example, do you feel you aren't loveable or are being ignored?

What are your core beliefs about your
relationship and about yourself?

What are your unresolved painful memories?

What is the worst possible outcome you can imagine
for the relationship that is causing you jealousy and
how could you resolve to live with that?

What do you need in your relationship to feel safe without needing
to control your partner? For example, do you need date nights or
positive affirmation and reassurance? Think practically and concretely.

What can you do to treat yourself like a valuable person?

If you were to adapt a rational and healthy story
about yourself, your relationship, and the cause of the
jealousy within it, what would that story be?

Wenzel also talks about retroactive jealous feelings. These occur "when
people feel jealous of their significant other's past sexual experiences and
relationships." This includes "comparing the number of your own past
partners, and the quality and quantity of sex with those partners, and your
current partner's sexual and relationship history."[16]

In order to heal jealousy, focus on expanding and shoring up your
self-esteem. Work on yourself, build your confidence. If you are having
real trouble dealing with your emotions, see a therapist for further support.

But don't ignore your intuition. If talking with your partner isn't helping, your jealousy might be warranted. Your partner could be cheating.
Ask yourself the following questions and try not to make assumptions
before you process things.

Questions to Ask:

What are my major concerns?

Is my partner open to change?

Are we working on things together?

WHEN YOUR PARTNER IS JEALOUS

Dealing with a jealous partner can be difficult, but patience and kindness are important. Find a way to listen, validate, and empathize with their emotions. Be honest about your own behaviors and what you might have done to trigger their fears. If you need to change things in your agreement, identify the parameters and talk about how they might not be working. Discuss new ideas and create an updated open monogamy agreement by going through the monogamy continuum exercise again.

Questions to Ask:

What is upsetting for you about our recent experiences?

What are some things that make you uncomfortable?

What do you think we should change?

What do you see for our future?

WHY THE TRUTH CAN SET YOU FREE

Open monogamy is ideologically aligned with honesty. Being open and honest is the basis for this kind of perpetual attempt at truth. It also means that as your needs change, you will have to be open about what you want. If you don't stand up for what you want, you can't blame your partner for what is not working or what you aren't getting.

It's not their fault if you aren't telling them what you want. It's time to speak your truth. Avoiding a potential argument that hasn't happened is a waste of energy.

You may want to change things in your marriage but have been afraid to start the conversation. You might have been worried it would hurt your partner so you've kept your feelings inside. By doing this, you may have created your own *monogamy trap*. You want to be with your partner and you don't want to cheat, but you want something more open. Sharing your feelings is the first step.

It can be hard to confront the truth. Using the skills you have learned so far in this book, you can articulate your desires. If you don't talk, it's almost impossible for your partner to read your mind. If you keep your needs repressed, you will continue to feel stuck and may be depriving yourself of the freedom that lies just outside of your own self-imposed marital constraints.

STAGES OF SEXUAL AND ROMANTIC RELATIONSHIPS

Just as we move through individual developmental stages, our partnerships grow and develop. In each stage, our agreements may need to be reviewed or updated. We renew our driver's license every couple of years, why not renew our monogamy agreement?

The stages of relationship follow a pattern that sociologists, anthropologists, and researchers say begins with a romantic love phase that eventually flattens out to a more companionate phase. This companionate stage has less passion, but more comfort. This familial phase is less erotic, but safe. For some couples it can lead to boredom, for others it can be the beginning of exploration outside the marriage. If a couple can stay together through the exploration and curiosity phases, they may outlast the inert phases of long-term partnership or skip right over the boredom to create the passion they desire.

I describe the phases of a relationship below using ten stages that every couple goes through, beginning with attraction and longing and ending with differentiation and separation. You can see that these stages can happen over the lifetime of a relationship, or they can be seen in a microcosm of a lifetime and may happen over a weekend. Often, these ten stages can occur over the course of an argument.

In an open relationship, you may find yourself in these stages with multiple partners. It is doubtful that you will be at the same stage with all your partners at the same time. Once you recognize the stage you are in, you can use this insight as a tool to talk honestly with your partner about what you are going through, what you are experiencing, and how to deal with the dilemmas and challenges of each relationship stage.

For instance, Lamika and Kai are in the communication phase. They had gone through conflict and felt alienated from one another, but curiosity about the other person's feelings had brought them back together and they talked through their separateness until they found they could empathize with each other. That communication allowed them to create changes in their relationship. They recognized that they wanted different things. This is where they are today. It is clear that they have been through these phases before, coming through differentiation and separateness and back to longing and attraction.

Stages of Relationships:

1. **Longing/Attraction:** When there is an attraction for the other, curiosity is still in place, and there is space to long for connection.

2. **Pursuing/Conquering:** A time of more intense longing and erotic connection through the first sexual experiences.

3. **Passion/Romance:** A time of erotic foundation that will preserve the relational connection later on in the relationship.

4. **Connection/Attachment:** The romantic love stage continues, usually lasting between three and twenty-seven months, leading to feelings of attachment and safety.

5. **Commitment/Relaxation:** Feeling securely attached and safe with a decrease of impression monitoring and focus on appearance. Both partners reveal more of their true self.

6. **Regression/Parentification:** Regress to an understanding of long-term, unconditional love, which is usually parental love. Partners become parentified, enter the power struggle stage and conflicts begin. Cognitive dissonance and emotional reactivity heightens.

7. **Conflict/Alienation:** The choice to end a relationship or disengage and refocus on outside interests. This stage includes maintenance sex or no sex, safety over eroticism, shut down or withdrawal, trauma to eroticism, affairs, betrayal, anger, or separation. Partners are in fight, flight, or freeze mode to protect themselves and the relationship.

8. **Curiosity/Empathy:** The waking up stage where one or both partners realize that there is a problem and choose to seek help or create a new form of relationship. Often includes reevaluating the monogamy agreement.

9. **Communication/Change:** Starting new conversations and redistributing erotic energy.

10. **Differentiation/Separation:** Creating and accepting a new relationship, a new understanding of self, and seeing the self as a separate sexual person.

ELANA

I interviewed Elana, a sexuality educator and creator of a conference for people interested in open relationships. Elana, age thirty-five, has been practicing polyamory her whole life. She is currently in three relationships, a primary relationship with Bill, age forty-two, and a secondary relationship with Steve, age fifty. She seems to have cycled through all these developmental stages at different times in her relationships. She lives on a forty-acre ranch outside of Provost, Utah. When I spoke with Elana, it was a snowy day in March. During our video call, she showed me around her beautiful home.

We talked about the conference that she started over five years ago. The first year, there were over 100 people registered. In the fifth year, the conference was sold out.

"We had to cancel it, just today," she said, "due to the outbreak of the COVID-19 coronavirus."

"Has that put all of your events on hold?" I asked.

"We have stopped all in-person events for now, due to COVID-19," she said. "My fear is that it will be like HIV, in that HIV had such a chilling effect. It's one of our main fears, our fear of death. I think that fear of our own death is destroying us. We are on high alert constantly because of social media. Our brains stay inflamed. Our connective tissue and autoimmune disorders are caused by that fear. And that fear is driving us away from each other."

Elana has been married for ten years and in her other relationship for over a decade. Both men have had other partners. At one point, Elana had a female partner.

"We were in a quad, a five-person group, but when I met Bill, I stopped going to see her and we became primary. Steve became primary with someone else on the coast," she said. "Bill and I have dated women and a couple and a gay man. Right now, Bill is dating one other person and we see another couple together; we consider them a sensual relationship. I also have a new girlfriend."

Elana defines herself as polyamorous with a "strong primary partner orientation."

"I like commitment," she said. "I like interdependency. I have these two long-term partners. Bill is my husband; he meets my deep need for romance and intimacy as well as domestic partnership."

She continued, "I put myself in the middle of a freedom/ security continuum. It's a perceived desire for security versus freedom and there is a mix of that. I have a certain amount of freedom and the cost of that freedom is security. You can't have equal amounts of security and freedom."

I asked Elana, "Have you always known that this is who you were? Have you always felt this about yourself?"

She said, "I grew up in a hippie family. They were way ahead of the curve. My parents got married on the beach in a hippie ceremony. The maid-of-honor slept with them that night. They had a variety of lovers that lived with us growing up. When I met my first husband at age sixteen, we started in an open relationship. We were together for ten years. I wanted other people but I was still very much in love with him."

She continued, "In my second marriage, I was monogamous for seven years. I was thirty-five years old. I found God and joined the Catholic church. I got religion and went straight and monogamous. That was my truth in that moment. During those seven years we raised kids and had businesses. But at one point, I identified that I was bisexual and wanted to have fun, sexy experiences. But it wasn't for him. We tried to do it for four years. He eventually decided it wasn't for him. After that, we knew it wasn't going to work."

"What is the most difficult part, or the most challenging part, of your relationships today?" I asked her.

"Bill's style of nonmonogamy is that he wants to do everything together. He defines it as monogamish. But Steve is grandfathered into our agreement and that is hard for Bill. It's hard for him when I go away with Steve. Steve and I have a beautiful relationship in a lot of ways, he supports me in my work but he doesn't have the family vibe that Bill and I have. Bill has trouble with Steve. Sometimes it's hard for him; we have disagreements about some of our decisions."

She continued, "My husband grew up with married parents. He was monogamous in his previous fourteen-year marriage. He is a therapist now and works with polyamorous and LGBTQIA+ people. When we fell in love it was like this wild hippie woman meets the stable guy. He lived on a cul-de-sac and I was a sex positive, poly, hippie sex worker. Now, Bill and I co-teach and do the sex positive thing together."

"How would Bill describe your relationship?" I asked.

"If you asked Bill, he would probably say that he enjoys the playful, sensual, sexual connection with others, and that it augments our relationship. Deepening our connection with others makes us closer. He doesn't want a significant other."

I asked, "Do you renew your agreements often?"

"The problem with agreements," she said, "is that each person has a different understanding of the agreement. A lot of the time they come from fear or are agreed to under duress."

"So, you don't have agreements?"

"We just take the pulse of the relationship, of how we are doing, and say if we have the bandwidth right now to have the upset or difficulty that might arise in our nervous system or in our bodies. At times he feels okay to be more playful, sensual, sexy, and at other times I can see that I don't want to, I can back up my own desire to meet him where he is."

"It sounds like you are constantly readjusting your agreement, taking the pulse of the relationship to see how you are doing, asking if you have the bandwidth to do whatever?"

"We both want each other to do the thing that brings the most authenticity of expression. If I can't handle that at the time, then it's up to me what I want to do in this relationship. Every time I have agreed to this or that, even if I go back and say let's change this agreement, it hasn't gone well. You can't just change it arbitrarily. Do we keep living by what we lived by before?

"What is the cost benefit analysis? What do I have to pay to get that? If it means that I have to be less slutty or less affectionate, I am willing to do that because I want their affection, time, or energy. If I decide to spend that time, affection, or energy, it's up to me."

"So, it's not arbitrary," I said. "You discuss it. What is the most meaningful part of your relationship for you?"

Elana said, "I have access to more facets of myself than if I was only with one person. If I was only with one person, these parts would be unmet. Bill brings out facets of myself and Steve meets facets of myself that Bill wouldn't. If I can love these two and have a deeper connection, then they can love more too. My orientation is toward love. Love is the biggest reason for all of this."

CHAPTER NINE

Aligning With Your True Values

Today, many of us are fumbling toward a new definition of monogamy. You may be too. And sometimes you may fail. In open relationships, as in closed ones, issues that come up are usually, at their foundation, a conflict around values. If all the partners involved have similar values and are operating from the same foundation, most conflicts can be worked through with healthy communication. Discovering what your values are and aligning with them means finding your own true north and lining up with your integrity. As you open your relationship, you must stay true to your values. This will help you when you feel stressed. Relationships are challenging, and with more personalities involved, they become even more interesting.

THE PRACTICAL VALUE OF SHARED VALUES

Molly and Jade live in a small town in Northern Maine. Jade is in marketing and works from home, Molly owns a local bicycle shop. They agreed to be interviewed about their open monogamy. I met with them over Zoom while they were sheltering in place during the pandemic.

Molly and Jade are both bright, articulate, older women who have been together for over forty years. They are in their seventies now and as a bi-racial couple they find that living in a small town has its challenges and its benefits. They got married in 2013 when the IRS made it possible to file jointly as a couple, even though it was still illegal for two women to marry in their state at the time.

Jade describes their open relationship as, "it depends," and "it needs explanations."

I asked her to clarify what she meant. She said, "The reality is that my spouse also has another relationship. I don't, but it's not out of the realm of possibility."

I asked her how she felt about their current arrangement. She said, "It works fine for now. Our life is lovely."

While talking with Molly and Jade, what struck me was their strong alignment in their shared and personal values. Although their arrangement is not perfect and they face prejudices due to their cultural backgrounds living in a primarily white area, they have created a family that works for them. They constantly return to what is important to both of them: transparency. Even when it isn't possible, they go back again and again to the significance of honesty above all else, and the freedom to live the life that works for them.

I asked Molly, "Do you define your relationship as polyamorous?"

Molly said, "A label is a way to hand someone an assumption you can live with."

I asked her, "How would you describe your relationship?"

She said, "I wouldn't pick the label polyamory. I don't think the idea of polyamory applies to me. I didn't set out to do this on purpose. I'm just me being me. I've lived long enough to know that this is what I want. Plus, people assume that being in this kind of relationship means you are promiscuous. This is far from the truth. Being open doesn't create promiscuity. I have just never wanted there to be rules."

Molly explained that she is married to Jade and has a long-term boyfriend on the side. He is very important to her and has been in her life for over thirty years. Jade has always known about him and has grown to like him. She isn't jealous or threatened by their relationship.

I asked them both if other people outside of their marriage knew about their unique arrangement.

Molly said, "I am not 'out.' My male partner is not 'out.' But it's not my story to tell. It's not my intention, it just worked out this way."

I asked, "How did you both come up with an agreement about having him as part of your marriage, or come up with an agreement about this arrangement? You are monogamous with each other, and with this other person, correct?"

Molly said, "When I got together with Jade, I said, 'Honestly, I'm not sure this is the last time I'm gonna fall in love. I might want others as well.'"

Jade looked at her and said, "Molly asked me what I thought of polyamory when we first met. I was sort of stunned, but I wasn't opposed to the idea. I had come from another relationship with someone who was convinced that I was monogamous and that this would be a problem for them. She assumed that because I was a lesbian, and most lesbians are monogamous, that I would never be okay with an open relationship. When she broke up with me, she kind of used that as an excuse. So, when Molly told me right up front that she was poly, and she explained what it was, I was ready to talk about it."

Molly said, "We met through a personal ad. When I told her 'I can't promise I'll be monogamous,' she seemed okay with it."

Jade said, "When we moved in, we had a lot of conversations about monogamy. Molly told me the truth; she wouldn't ever close her mind to being in another relationship."

Molly said, "Jade and I had a small wedding on the cliffs. We wrote our own vows. Our vows never said anything about being monogamous. We said, 'I take you as my partner, lover, and friend,' not death do us part."

Jade added, "Our vows were intentional and serious. We spent a long time hammering out what we were agreeing to, and also what we were not agreeing to, and what we were building."

Molly said, "We were both in the same place, that our relationship was not going to be totally traditional monogamy. But nothing happened for a while. ThenI met a guy. I was so surprised to have that feeling. It was a friendship at first and it grew slowly over a couple of years. I thought it would go away. I told Jade everything. She said she didn't feel threatened by Tom. It took a long time before anything happened."

Jade said, "I was her ally all along the way. I had feelings about how things were going to proceed." She looked at Molly and then at me, "Molly kept asking me, 'How is this for you? If you are against it, I would consider not doing it.'"

"Did you have rules?" I asked.

Jade said, "I told Molly I would rather not be present when they were holding hands or kissing. Today, we are past that. So many years have gone by."

Molly said, "When Tom spends the night it's not an issue because we sleep together in my room, he sleeps with me."

Jade said, "For some years, Molly and I have had separate bedrooms. I have a home office for my work. Molly and I sleep together sometimes, but we have always wanted our own spaces, since we first moved in together."

"It's worked out," Molly said.

Jade said, "I told Molly at first that I didn't want to be in the house when she and Tom were being sexual. We worked it out that I would go on errands and let her know when I was going to come home. That didn't last that long."

I said, "Wow, so at first you didn't want to be around them when they were being affectionate, but eventually were okay with sleepovers?"

Jade said, "All of that developed over time. Now, he spends one night a week here—Thursday nights. Molly always made me feel prioritized with no intent of leaving me or getting married to him. So, it just didn't threaten our relationship."

DATING SOMEONE CLOSED

Other couples do it differently. When I asked Tom how he and his wife manage their relationship with Molly and Jade, he said, "I think we have a good thing, but we are not totally open. I am, but she's not. She knows about my relationship. But we have a don't ask, don't tell relationship. She doesn't like it, but it's a significant relationship in my life, and she knows it. Once in a while there is a need to talk; and she ok with it, she is not against the whole thing."

"How have you managed during the shelter-in-place restrictions," I asked. "Has it been more difficult with your wife?"

Tom said, "We talked about it right away when COVID-19 hit. We talk about it all the time still. I think she is fine with it, but she doesn't want to know any details. I asked her if she wants a boyfriend, but she says it's too much trouble. Sometimes she comes with me and we all eat dinner together. She really likes Molly and Jade, they all get along. I think she would rather stay home and be with our dogs; she seems happy."

I asked what happens when you get together, now that COVID is a real thing? "We want to protect each other," Molly said. "We all had a conversation about this. We needed a plan for protection against COVID. I guess a lot of people did that. I asked Tom if he thought our plan was safe, if we should be six feet apart when we saw each other. He said his wife was fine with it, so we all agreed it was okay to be in our safe pod together."

"It seems like you were all really honest and wanted to talk about it," I said.

"Yes," Molly said. "He even told her, 'I think we should merge households, to be safe.' But she didn't all want to live together. It's nice to have our houses in different parts of Maine; they have one right on the water and we have one in the woods."

"So, what is your agreement now?" I asked.

"Our agreement now," Molly said, "is that we are all honest with each other. We talk about how we feel and what we want. His wife isn't interested in seeing other people, but she is fine with our arrangement."

Jade said, "We are extremely transparent and intentional. We are actually helping each other grow in that respect. We are pushing growth in our marriage, which has improved since we have all been together. Tom and his wife talk more than they ever have. Our priority is honesty. He has gotten much more open and honest with all of us since this all started. It's helped."

"So, your open marriage has improved Tom's closed marriage?" I asked.

Jade said, "Well, yes, in many ways. We are all open now, we all talk and things are friendly and transparent. She comes over for dinner and we like each other, as a foursome. We don't have sex with each other, but we are all friends."

I asked both Molly and Jade, "What is the most challenging part of all of this?"

Molly said, "For me, it's Tom's role in my life. He wants more sometimes. He is confused about being my boyfriend and his role I think."

Jade said, "That is one of the hardest parts for me too. Who knows, maybe if his wife were more open and had her own relationship, or if I had someone else, it would be easier for everyone. But we are all accepting of it. I think everything could be more open and it would be easier. It's important to me that this is not screwed up. I don't want people to be hurt."

Molly said, "I appreciate Jade talking about the need to be honest. That is so important to me as well. I told Tom, I am never going to do the infidelity thing, so you should know that. So don't ever lie to me or to your wife. I like that we are all friends, we hang out, the four of us."

Jade said, "It can be hard for outside partners, for sure, if there is more intimacy between their partner and someone else than with them, don't you think?"

"I imagine sometimes she might feel jealous," I said. "Do you ever get jealous?" I looked at Jade.

She said, "I have been aware that I've felt a little jealous. As I sit here and sift through some feelings, I can be honest about that. After Tom's wife became aware of what was happening, there was tension. She found out and she was really upset. That was hard. I knew how she felt, but on the other hand, it was never a secret from me. Molly never kept it from me. Eventually they worked it out and we are all good friends now."

"Does it bother you that Molly and Tom are so close?" I asked.

Jade said, "It's actually good for me that they have that intimate relationship. I know Molly's happy. But it has been hard for me too. One weekend, Tom and another couple came over. I realized that everyone in the room was in more than one relationship, except for me. I was nervous. I had a vague fear that I was the odd person. Everyone was into talking about nonmonogamy and I thought to myself, do I want to be here?"

"Do you like Tom?" I asked Jade.

"I like him," Jade said. "We have a kind of sibling relationship, it's a sibling dynamic, it is sort of like that. We get each other's goat. He teases me. We get along really well.

COVID-Bonded

Safety was a dilemma for many people who wanted to stay connected in open relationships during the COVID-19 pandemic. Some people with outside partners chose to see each other and considered their outside partners part of their COVID families. These people are what I call *COVID-bonded* with their loved ones. COVID-bonded means that they have chosen to be with those they feel closest to and are aware of the risks. Some got together after being tested or after receiving an antibody test. Some waited until they were vaccinated. And some chose to practice safe distancing.

When a partner's spouse will not consent to be part of the COVID-bonded group, it can create stress among the whole system. Decisions have to be made about who will continue to have contact and what kind of contact that will include.

This can be a moral issue for many people, when the problem of spreading infection is divisive among family members and open monogamy groups.

WHO DO YOU TELL?

Leif and Eugenia, who we met earlier, are not "out" about their particular type of monogamy.

"Some people know," Leif said. "I would say we are 'quiet' but not 'closeted.' Eugenia has told her sister, even though she knows her sister is much less sexually open. Some of our friends know, and some of my coworkers."

When Leif's son was born, he decided he didn't want to lie to him or ask his son to lie for him if it came up. Children have a way of being honest, in unpredictable ways, and Leif didn't want to put pressure on him to have to explain his father's relationships with people. His son hasn't liked all of Leif's "friends," and Leif let him know that he has a say in whether they stuck around. The shared veto power made things easier.

"My wife, my son's mother, died when he was six. So, it was him and me for a long time. I had a girlfriend, and my son was close to her like he was to his mom. She had been around before my wife died and he was attached to her. I think poly can be good for kids. More loving adults to go around."

Involving or not involving kids can be a redline for some people. The decision to honor the secret of an open lifestyle or participate in the open discussion of an extended family is something that should be discussed in your open monogamy agreement and revisited as family members grow up and their needs and relationships change.

Discerning Your Values

This next exercise can help you begin to think about what is important to you. Your values are where your choices align with your behaviors, and this exercise can help you create your ideal vision for your future.

Questions to Ask Yourself:

What are my priorities?

What are the things that matter to me?

What do I believe in?

What do I stand for?

What do I want for my life?

If I could jump forward in time to an ideal place, where would I land?

What is important in a relationship?

How should children be raised?

How should the elderly be treated?

How do I want to be remembered?

○

IS OPEN MONOGAMY A FORM OF SEXUAL ORIENTATION?

Some people believe that being polyamorous is more than just a preference; they believe it is an orientation. Trying to be traditionally monogamous may feel like you are going against your own values, and even against who you are meant to be.

Sociological researcher Elisabeth "Eli" Sheff said it depends. Legally, polyamory is not a sexual orientation. Sexual orientation is a pattern of sexual, romantic, and emotional attraction and identity that is distinct from gender identity, which is the internal sense of being male, female, or nonbinary. Some people who define themselves as poly say that polyamory is an orientation. Sexual orientation is defined by who you desire for a partner. If you desire someone of the opposite sex, you are considered heterosexual; if you desire someone of the same sex, you are considered homosexual; and if you desire both, you are considered bisexual. Many people are more fluid in their attractions and don't like to be defined in any one category. Orientation can also be determined by your committed relationship.

I interviewed Sheff about what it means to be in a poly relationship. She said the basic ethical framework of poly is that it is based on honesty, self-respect, and owning up if you've made a mistake. She said, "Traditional monogamy has virtually no chance in contemporary society."

I asked, "Is nonmonogamy the future of marriage?"

She said, "Nonmonogamy is not paradise. People who are naturally monogamous are not going to be happy with a nonmonogamous partner. Trying to smash them into a nonmonogamous relationship can do them psychic harm."

She continued, "For some people, monogamy doesn't work. Some people are just nonmonogamous; they are hardwired for it, it's an orientation, they can't be in a monogamous relationship. It's like a desire for a partner of a specific gender. Sometimes it doesn't work. Deep romantic partnerships might not work, nonmonogamous mismatches can fall deeply in love. Some people are multiple by orientation and on that level, they don't match."

"Have you had personal experience with this?" I asked.

"I was in love with a man who wanted nonmonogamy; he really liked variety. Sexual variety doesn't signal dissatisfaction with your current partner, it may just mean they like variety and can't make that go away. It's hard-wired into some people. I am currently married to a woman. We each do our own thing. We follow our own rules. It's a closed, open relationship. It's gone great."

I asked her, "Is monogamy hardwired in some people as well?"

"Some want exclusivity. People at the edges of the scale are born that way. The vast majority fall in between. They might say, 'I don't want to share, but I'd love a harem, but not to share, only to focus on me.' If they are nonmonogamous by orientation, sharing is not painful. Losing resources or wanting more time may be painful, but the idea of their partner wanting sex with someone else is not painful. They can deal with jealousy and sustain nonmonogamy. Other people are more on the monogamous side and can find their sexual variety through fantasy. For other deeply monogamous people, looking at porn feels like cheating."

I asked her, "In your opinion, which is more beneficial, monogamy or nonmonogamy?"

She said, "There are advantages and disadvantages within the rubric. Nonmonogamy can help relationships be more durable. If we never agree to monogamy, we never have to hurt each other that way. You can maintain the strong bond without screwing up the relationship stuff and have sexual variety. Monogamy is difficult to maintain and hard to sustain and can be painful. When people break their monogamy, they are really hurt and devastated."

> If we never agree to monogamy, we never
> have to hurt each other that way.

She continued, "A single partnership is difficult to sustain; seventy years of having sex with no one else is a daunting prospect. Sex is tempting, it's everywhere."

It used to be easier to stick with just one partner. In the time of the pre-industrial revolution, a person met about three hundred people in their lifetime and were related to most of them.

"Unless you were royalty," Sheff said. "The wealthy have never truly been monogamous. Wealthy men have never been monogamous. The elite in power always had multiple women, wives, or mistresses. The wealthier population had affairs, and eventually that has trickled down to the non-wealthy. Now, women and people of all social classes have access to nonmonogamy because they can meet a wide variety of people."

I asked her, "What advice would you give couples today?"

Sheff said, "Be willing to explore alternatives. If you are both in the midrange of interest for nonmonogamy, meaning you have some desire and at the same time some reluctance to share, first figure out what is underlying the reluctance. If it's not reluctance for your partner to have sex with other people, it may be that you are worried it would take away resources from the family. In that case, swinging might work. You could allow sex but have a strong agreement about resources and don't break it."

"So, agree that each of you can have sex with other people, but talk about the division of time, attention, affection, things like that?" I asked.

"Yes," she said. "For others, they might just want to talk to people but not have sex with them. If eroticism is a big part of a person and it's painful to live without it, they could make it part of the relationship without the sex. It could be a *catch-and-release agreement*. The more erotic partner can flirt with others and grope and even make out on the dance floor, but no intercourse and no getting phone numbers. This allows for the fullness of eroticism but saves the sexuality for the partner. It only works if the partner can deal with that. There needs to be room for renegotiation."

"Anything else you can suggest?"

"Try it. If it doesn't work, it means you made an agreement that doesn't work."

FAMILY VALUES

One thing I have noticed in my private practice working with couples in open or polyamorous relationships is that groups of people who are in romantic partnerships create family bonds quite easily. Polyamorous pods or quads find that initially the comfort of more partners, more parents, more grown-ups, more lovers, and more people to clean and cook and provide comfort, affection, attention, and sex is wonderful. There is more to go around, more of everything. It feels like a big happy community. For some people, it feels like the family they never had; the intentional, connected, and healthy support system that can heal them from the dysfunctional childhood that they are trying to get away from. This in no way means that people who are attracted to poly come from dysfunctional families. It takes a high level of communication to manage one relationship, much less multiple relationships, so I wouldn't make a direct connection to dysfunctional childhoods leading to polyamory. However, anecdotally, what I do notice is that when people are in a big happy polyamorous family, they tend to act out their sibling roles.

They argue about who gets the best bedroom or the best bike or the most time or the most affection. Whatever their issues were in their childhood, whatever they felt deprived of, or however they acted out, shows up. This happens in monogamous relationships as well, but in a parentified way. We project our unmet needs onto our spouse or committed partner. We all choose someone who has the positive and negative traits of our caretakers. Initially, we project that this person will bring us everything we have ever looked for in a partner, and then they don't. We blame them for being somehow unworthy or not enough and we look elsewhere for what is, in truth, surely lacking in ourselves. We are looking for a mirror of what we need to heal from our past. This is true of all of us. We marry someone we are fundamentally and totally incompatible with in order to grow as human beings. It is a marvelous, albeit painful system.

With open monogamy, these issues become magnified. At first, it seems like the perfect answer to the age-old problem of trying to find one partner who can fulfill all our needs. We realize after the romantic phase of a relationship has worn off, that no one person can be our everything. So, we assume that having more than one partner can fulfill our needs and we get to stay with our first partner and continue what has been mostly working.

Yet, this is not a perfect answer. It bypasses the original problem, which is us. We will have to deal with our stuff in not only one relationship, but in two, or three, or more. And so, we are faced with our true selves, in multiple arenas, in multiple mirrors. There are many chances to prove ourselves worthy of love, to get it right, to find what we are missing. We are all destined to repeat our childhood until we get conscious about what we are doing.

For Molly, Jade, and Tom, the sibling teasing, the fight for time, and the protection of the outside partner can be traced back to their relationships with their brothers and sisters. There is nothing wrong with the majority of these interactions. Acting out sibling stuff does not have to be a curse; it is just something to consider.

In many families, however, there is rivalry, competition, or distance. Siblings fight and they compete for their parent's attention and love. They react to conflict by retreating and distancing themselves or by acting out and distracting everyone with their own drama, trying to hold their parents' marriage together by becoming the conflictual glue that will keep the family from splitting apart.

When a group of poly partners are together, it is bound to trigger everyone's past relationships. It can feel like one big Thanksgiving dinner from the past, and very few people had perfect pasts. The important thing here is to recognize what is happening for you as you open your monogamy. What were the values that you were taught in your family and how are they affecting you now?

Some family values are the basis of your whole moral structure. Others are insidious and destructive. Things like, "Big boys don't cry," or "Girls shouldn't have sex before marriage," are examples of the myriad of "values" that were placed on you and your siblings in childhood. Some values apply to gender roles, others to stereotypes around race and culture.

You also learned roles within your family. Are you the caretaker? The clown? The damaged one? Do you blame others, or do you take the blame? Are you the martyr? Are you the smart one? The introvert? How many of these roles are actually roles you want, and what are the roles you were pushed into as a child and you want to let go of?

Sibling Triggers

The sibling triggers cannot be helped. For some people, love that is divided among multiple partners is never enough. For others, it can feel adequate, but flawed.

Questions to Ask Yourself:

Were you given enough love as a child?

Were you given the time, attention, and affection you needed?

What do you feel you missed out on?

Did one of your siblings get more than you?

Were the resources spread around evenly?

These sibling issues will influence the kind and type of love you need in a relationship. You may project your needs for equality onto your primary partner or onto multiple partners, as if they were your parents or siblings.

Things to Think About:

Can any of our relationships, whether romantic, intimate, or sexual, ever be equal?

Are you feeling like your relationships are not fair?

Which of your relationships is a priority for you?

How do you share with outside partners?

How do you react when you don't receive the same attention as other partners?

Betrayal and hurt can stem from implicit expectations that are not discussed regarding time, attention, affection, and sex and how they are divided among partners. Things that are assumed in a relationship but never talked about or agreed upon can cause disappointment and misunderstanding.

Share with your partner how you feel about their outside relationships and what it brings up for you.

DEFINING YOUR SEXUAL VALUES

Your perception of sex was first learned in your family of origin. You learned what it means to be a man, a woman, gay, straight, bi, cis or trans, and what it means to be in a relationship. You learned what sex means and how to react when you have it or don't have it. You learned how other people react when you talk about it. You learned to talk about it or not talk about it. Those roles are deeply entrenched in your sense of self.

Then, you learn from your peers, social media, and from the outside world who you are, as it's reflected back to you as you grow into the person you are today. Your childhood, adolescence, and early adulthood determine whether you feel accepted, accept yourself, or feel excluded and how you determine what makes you feel sexual.

Your sexual values also determined the things that are important to you in your erotic life. They may or may not be the same as your partner's values, and, in fact, they may be totally opposite or different. You may seek an outside partner who shares your sexual values because you feel a mismatch with your current partner. Or you might want to share your sexual values with the partner you have and talk more about what they mean to you. Have a conversation. Start with your own definitions and then ask about your partner's values.

This next exercise will help you define your sexual values and can be the beginning of a conversation about what you want in an erotic relationship. Rate the values and share with your partner.

Sexual Values

GOAL: To learn about your sexual values and increase connection with your partner.

DIRECTIONS: You can do this alone or with a partner. It is recommended that you try this alone first and then share the list with your partner.

Go down the list and number each value according to how important it is for you, going from 1 (not so important) to 5 (very important)

Safety ____	Passion ____
Trust ____	Adventure ____
Connection ____	Kink ____
Intensity ____	Romance ____
Challenge ____	Tension ____
Fantasy ____	Variety ____
Fear ____	Honesty ____
Thrill ____	Consent ____
Comfort ____	

Talk about your list and what each value means to you.

◡

Given your values, what is going to be important to you in your open monogamy? You can decide what you want as you go along, or you can think about the many configurations and combinations that are available to you. Going back to the monogamy continuum, remember that there are many options within each category. For instance, if you and your partner agree, and you have the energy, you can have your primary relationship and have one outside relationship, like Molly and Jade's arrangement. They are exclusive with Tom, and Tom does not have any partners outside of his wife with whom he is not sexual.

You could have a primary partnership and each have an outside partner, making it a foursome. You could share these partners and only see them when you are together. You could each be sexual with them or romantically involved, depending on if you want to be with those outside partners together, or separately.

POLYFIDELITY

People who are in a *polyfidelity relationship agreement* believe fidelity is an important value and choose to be faithful to their group of partners. They have a specific, multi-partner relationship agreement and if one of the partners goes outside of the group, it is a betrayal to the whole group.

VALUING EACH OTHER

Danny and Alfred have been in a thruple for six years and married for over twenty years. They chose to open their relationship to include a younger man, someone they met online. Chad was fourteen years younger than both of them. He was biracial, which was important for Danny who had grown up being bullied in his all-white neighborhood for being gay and Black. Alfred was older than Danny and an accomplished oboe player in the New York Philharmonic. He was a white, Jewish, gay man who had recently recovered from prostate cancer.

Danny and Alfred had never been with other men during their marriage, but they agreed that when Chad came along, they would make an exception.

Danny said, "Chad makes me feel young, he doesn't treat me like a 'daddy' which I hate, and since Alfred's surgery, well, it's nice to have a young man's erection."

I asked Alfred how he felt about that.

Alfred said, "Since my prostate surgery, sex hasn't been the same for me. It's still important that Danny and I spend intimate time together, but I just don't have the desire, nor the capability that I used to. I think Chad is the answer."

Chad moved into their Upper West Side penthouse in Manhattan and had been living there for almost five years. The three of them identified as being in a thruple, which Danny said worked fine for him.

"Chad will never replace Alfred; he is my husband and the love of my life. But Chad is fun in bed and fills that need. He knows his place and we can take care of him. He needs our support right now. He needed a green card, and we could help him with his immigration. We are using each other, but in a loving, supportive, family way. But not in a daddy way," he laughed.

"Does Chad feel like he is here voluntarily or does he feel like he has to be here?" I asked.

Alfred said, "Oh, he says he loves being here. Who wouldn't? We give him everything he wants, the sex is great, and he gets to live a lifestyle that he would never get to experience. We take him to the theater and to the symphony, and we buy him clothes. Yes, we take care of him. So? He takes care of us. We love each other."

"Do you think your values align?" I asked.

Alfred said, "We care about each other's well-being, we are there for each other, we trust each other, and I think those are important values: caring, trust, and being there. We aren't swingers."

ARE SWINGERS HAPPIER?

Studies show that people who have more open relationships report happier marriages, in general. Twenty-seven percent of those surveyed say that *swinging* strengthened their marriage, made their relationships happier, and made the sex at home more satisfying.

By going outside the marriage, they were able to express more affection and had better communication with their spouse. They reported less anxiety and depression than the general population. And, counterintuitively, they expressed less jealousy than monogamous couples. But swinging is not for everyone.

Swinging is a type of open relationship where both partners may or may not be together when they have sexual experiences with outside relationships. The term "swinging" goes back to the 1970s when it was made prevalent in popular culture, but fewer people define their open relationships in this way. Alfred, Danny, and Chad originally described themselves as swingers, but then found the term too cliché. They found that the term thruple better identified their unique relationship. They are monogamous to their thruple and don't plan on going outside of their threesome to "swing" although they discuss the relationship on a regular basis and are open to change if any of the three of them become unhappy.

"Danny might want someone else eventually," Alfred said. "For now, this works for us. I know some people don't understand us, but that's okay."

MARRIAGE AND METAMOURS

For some, opening the marriage can complicate a stable relationship. Despite the reputation gay men have for being in open relationships, many gay male couples stay monogamous. For Alfred and Danny, their relationship is based on polyfidelity. They have been tempted to open it to other men, but said, "It would change our relationship and it seems like a lot of work."

Danny said, "There are some things that are sacred. We don't do certain things with Chad. We keep certain sex acts between Al and me only. I've seen other men who open it all up, I mean, I lived through the AIDS epidemic and look where that got us. I am cautious. We are all on PrEP (pre-exposure prophylaxis)[1] and it's fine now, but I'm not going to hook up with just anybody. We aren't swingers. We are exclusive, just the three of us."

Alfred said, "We are metamours. I don't have sex with Chad, but Danny does. So, he is my metamour and I am his. It sounds complicated, but to us, it works."

As we learned in chapter two, a metamour is a partner who . . . is not a lover themselves. They can be bonded, and consider themselves to be in a polyamorous relationship or in a poly family, but there is no sexual relationship. For Alfred, his approval as a metamour is crucial to the survival of the thruple, even if Chad and Danny are the only ones who are currently sexual.

"This was always a fantasy of Danny's, to be in a threesome. I just never thought we'd be doing it for this long," Alfred said.

"Did you want this too?" I asked.

"Well, yes, of course, but it's more for Danny."

Danny said, "Wait, Alfred, this is working for you, too, isn't it? I don't want to feel like I'm coercing anyone."

"No, of course not," Alfred said. "We check in all the time. If there is ever a time when I don't want to do it anymore, or Chad can't give his consent, or we feel we are blocking him from another relationship with someone his own age, we would back off and let him go, of course."

"This is not an ownership thing. We love him," Danny said. "But our marriage will always come first, that's the reality."

SPIRITUAL VALUES

For all the couples and individuals I interviewed for this book and the hundreds of people I have worked with who have struggled to open their monogamy, the journey itself has been the challenge, as well as the joy. Having the courage to confront what is not working in their relationship and focus instead on the strengths in their bond has taught my clients many lessons. The most important thing they have all learned is that having an open relationship is a spiritual journey.

What constitutes a spiritual journey? Every spiritual journey has identifiable stages. There is a search for meaning, there are dark confusing times where no meaning can be found, there are moments of enlightenment when you realize you have a purpose, and there is a realization that there is some operating force greater than you. A spiritual journey takes you on a path that requires you to let go of your own egoic needs and shows you that you are here to help others and that all there really is, is love. And the more you

With an open monogamy relationship, there is a struggle to grow out of the limitations one has put oneself under, the small world you have crowded yourself into because of self-imposed limitations and restrictions. With that, there comes a search for more. Because this is not an individual journey, but a journey with a partner, the search for meaning can be lonely and hard, it can be a power struggle rife with conflict, it can be intimate and connecting, and it can bring you to a new awakened place of true enlightenment where you realize your place, your shared purpose, is to help each other grow. This type of relationship leaves no room for cowardice. There is only the continued search for meaning and a perpetual battle for truth. Couples who dare to take on this challenge will find meaning in each challenge, in each struggle, and will seek to find clarity by continuously pushing to understand. These are the steps toward enlightenment. It is not a smooth path.

If you are on this path, you will feel like many couples do. You will find yourself lost, lonely, and in the proverbial dark night of the soul—the stuck place where you believe nothing will ever work, where a choice must be made, and where you might have to lose it all. And yet, you may find that if you stick to your values and are truthful and loving, you come through those dark places and discover light on the other side.

When you make space for truth, there is more room for joy and more places to find happiness and play.

What Constitutes a Spiritual Journey?

Search for meaning

Dark confusing times

Moments of enlightenment

Finding purpose

Realization of a greater force

Letting go of egoic needs

Desire to help others

Realizing all is love

Giving love creates more love

SPIRITUAL GUILT

Many of us have been brought up with religious beliefs that have their roots in shame and guilt. Like the belief that having all you want is selfish, or bad, or will lead to no good. This belief is so strong in us that it infiltrates everything. To some extent, it acts as an important spiritual boundary. Not wanting everything and letting go of want and desire can decrease the incredible pain of wanting, of never having, and of always seeking and searching for what you don't have.

But the guilt around seeking pleasure is rampant. We are taught that wanting pleasure is either sinful or indulgent, and so we either avoid it because we feel guilty, or we binge on it and then feel remorse and hungover afterward. We fear we'll be punished for experiencing too much pleasure and sometimes we even build in our own sabotage to ensure punishment, to make sure we don't get away with too much.

Shame and guilt are a trap. They can be a way to hold yourself hostage, to prevent yourself from getting the emotional, sexual, and romantic pleasure you deserve in your life.

SACRED PLEASURE

Reframe your sexuality as a part of your spirituality. A spiritual open monogamy means you can expand on the pleasure you experience now and give and receive more. Think about pleasure with the purpose of discovering more of who you are and more of who your partner could be. In this way, you might share and explore a wider range of relationships so that the two of you can become loving partners with more to share. This doesn't mean you don't have limits. Ask yourself the following:

What Are Our Limits?

What is sacred between us?

What is the most pleasurable thing I can imagine?

What do I want and believe I can share with others?

How can our happiness influence those around us?

What is the meaning of our love?

Your open monogamy agreement should be intentional, consensual, and joyful. Honor what is sacred between you and trust that your love will flow out to others.

Now that you are ready and have the strength to begin, I wish you the best of luck and much joy along your open monogamy journey. I know things may be bumpy at times, but the truth will set you free—free of the lies, fears, and hurt that can come from hiding who you truly are.

Have fun with it. Life is supposed to be a good time. Go forth and play. Spread love and kindness. Be good to one another.

Send pics.

CONCLUSION

The Future of Marriage

"If you want to understand the universe, you have to
understand energy, vibration, and frequency."

NIKOLA TESLA

The definition of marriage has changed. We are changing it. How
will we define it fifty or one hundred years from now? Will marriage,
as we know it, even exist in the future?

Right now, it takes two people to get married, but only one person
to end it. Divorce is the legal dissolution of a partnership and the end
of a contract.

The whole idea we have about trying to "find the right person" is a recipe
for failure. Our deep cultural belief in romantic partnership is based on
the search for a soulmate. The idea that we all have a soulmate out there
implies that there is one ideal person for each of us. But when we find that
one perfect person, marry them, and then that relationship ends, we have
to rewrite the whole history of our soulmate relationship and think to
ourselves, "Well, that was a mistake, that couldn't have been my soulmate."
Then we have to start over and begin the search again, this time hoping to
find our true soulmate.

Could it be, instead, that everyone we meet is our soulmate? Perhaps we
travel in soul packs and learn from every person we come across in our lifetime. We learn from every partner, whether we are together for a night or a
decade. We are also soulmates with every coworker, every child, every au-
thority figure, every friend, and everyone we run into at the grocery store.

Elisabeth "Eli" Sheff studied poly families for over twenty years and found that children raised in poly groups were more likely to feel free to choose their own type of relationship format as they aged, open or traditional. They were also more likely to value honesty, openness, communication, and togetherness. They appreciated that there were always other children to play with when they were growing up, and their one complaint was that there were also a lot of adults, so they could never get away with anything.

Perhaps we are moving from the individual idea of love to a group or village perspective. Maybe it does take a village to raise a family. Particularly when we are all working; identify as male, female, gay, and straight; don't adhere to traditional gender roles; and recognize that the more parental figures in a child's life, the better. As we have moved away from living with our extended families in one home, we have isolated our children from their experience of multiple parents and grandparents. During the pandemic, families were separated from their elders, afraid to include them in family gatherings, and fearful that their health would be at risk. Now, post pandemic and post quarantine, we realize the importance of family more than ever. Moving to a poly-partner monogamy may actually foster more support for children.

We will also see the expansion of the definition of "parent." Couples are waiting until later than ever before to have children and many women are freezing their eggs, putting off childbearing. Fertility treatments, egg donors, surrogate parenting with IVF, and hormone treatments are more popular than ever, which means that the definition of parenting will expand as well.[1]

Children reared in packs, with alternate parents and grandparents, will have exposure to a variety of experiences and opinions, with caregivers that range in age from twenty to ninety. With more families living in village-like arrangements, childcare is expanded to cover more needs and involves more people who can contribute their skills, interests, and aptitudes to the home. There will be more community resources and all members can work toward the reclaiming of our planet.

In the future, with monogamy arrangements becoming more fluid and flexible, the likelihood that there will be options for open marriages makes sense. Couples will have more open sexual agreements, polyamory will be more common, and perhaps federal law will eventually follow in the footsteps of Cambridge and recognize the partnership rights of non-nuclear families.

With the fluidity of sexual orientation and identity, more people will be androgynous and there will be less of a focus on gender. There will be more people who identify as trans, with more fluid or bisexual identifying than ever before. Some say there will be more intersex and asexual babies who are born without a clear gender identity. There is no way to prove this. However, it is possible that parents will not be so quick to choose surgery to assign a sex when it is physically ambiguous. We will judge a person less on their sexual identity and more on how they treat others.

Right now, about 40 percent of Americans think marriage as a concept is obsolete. They are not sure if the legal aspect of marriage is even necessary. As a result, fewer couples than ever before are married, and marriage rates will continue to decline into the future. There is no longer a motivation to legally marry; couples don't need to marry to have children, to pass on their property, or to have sex. In one hundred years, marriage as we know it may not even exist.

Humans, however, will always want to partner up. Partnering is a basic human propensity. We love to fall in love. We love to have a special person or another someone with whom we feel a deep, emotional, and spiritual connection.

In the future, could we have this deep, spiritual connection with many partners, not just one? How many soulmates could we have in one lifetime?

ALTERNATIVE RELATIONSHIPS ARE THE FUTURE

Being in an open monogamy is like gathering wool; it doesn't matter how many sheep you have, what matters is what you do with the wool. Do you keep it in a pile, do you make nice sweaters, do you throw it away? In other words, how do you manage your open monogamy, how do you give it enough room to grow and change and develop over time, while checking in often enough with your partner about boundaries?

EDWARD AND SCOTT

Edward, author of three books on gay erotica, and his husband Scott, an architect and designer, have an open relationship where "the key is to make the fantasy real."

Edward said, "We make our fantasies real, but we are always responsible for each other."

Scott is sixty-four with a solid build, dark eyes, and salt-and-pepper hair. Edward is sixty-two and tall and lanky, with silver hair. Both men exercise regularly, walk their dogs in their small New England neighborhood in the afternoon, and "play with their friends" on the weekend. They have been married for thirty-four years, since they were very young, and before gay marriage was legal. I asked them to talk with me about their open monogamy agreement.

Edward said, "When people hear 'open' monogamy, they might hear the word 'open' first and think that means being open to everything. I suppose that's what makes the idea of 'open monogamy' distinctive. But for us, everything begins and ends with our monogamy. The strength of our relationship is based on that key factor. Our monogamy allows us to invite other people into our lives, sexually and romantically. Since we only play together, we only do things when we are each in the room. It's for our relationship, it's for us. Our way of doing this works for us, because it's for Scott and me. We believe it really is about opening our marriage to others. We let them in, it's a momentary thing, we let them in just to play. Our relationship, our commitment, is the anchor. It's the basis of trust and honor we need in order to share our intimacy with others. It was just us two in the beginning and it will be just us two in the end."

Is this the future of relationships? Our primary monogamy will grow so strong that it will allow for expansion? For more love than ever before?

MAYBE WE NEED TO GROW UP

Right now, we are marrying later than ever, delaying commitment, and putting off child-rearing. Could it be that because we are living longer than ever before, we aren't "settling down" with one person until later in life and waiting to grow up? Maybe we are staying in a sort of adolescent stage of emotional development, choosing to date a bunch of people instead of committing to marriage. Maybe we want to have multiple partners and are avoiding the real work of being with one partner. Maybe open relationships are the ultimate manifestation of ADD; we can't pay attention to one person long enough to make it work. Perhaps we are so divisive in our attention span that we get bored and move on too fast. Perhaps we are in a perpetual state of adolescence; we just want more sex, more fun, and fewer responsibilities.

Or maybe we have learned to be multi-attentive. Since we live in a society that demands our attention in multiple ways from the time we are born, perhaps our brains have developed in a way that allows us focus on more than one person at a time. Maybe kids that have been raised with their headphones on while playing video games really are able to be divisive in their attention.

What does this mean for us later in life? Are we all simply developmental adolescents until the last quarter century of our lives when we finally settle down into adulthood and choose one partner to live happily ever after with only because we are just too tired to keep up the pace? Or maybe with better medicine and health care we will have more energy to keep it all up.

TECHNOLOGY

With the advance of technology, more people may choose to integrate virtual reality, artificial intelligence, and robotic sex into their daily lives. Many couples will have long-distance relationships and use teledildonics to stay connected. Already, pornography and interactive webcam sex has become a way to maintain monogamy. It creates variety without adding an extra real-life partner. These computerized digital experiences are accessible and virtually realistic, making them interactive enough to keep living-apart-together (LAT) relationships connected and passionate. Virtual dolls that use robotics and artificial intelligence are increasingly available to the public and prices have become more reasonable. These sex robots have primarily been marketed to men but can be used by couples. They are interactive and, in many ways, empathic sexual partners.

But even our most advanced future scientific developments will not be able to replace the intimate emotional and physical connection between real people. The spiritual dimension of a relationship cannot be replaced with a robot. However, with viruses and sexually transmitted infections (STIs), we may have to measure the risks and rewards of open relationships with multiple partners. Testing will have to be more mobile and accessible, with home STI tests and perhaps viral kits as well.

My hope is that in the not-so-distant future all sexuality will be seen as healthy and no longer a threat to our relationships. Sex will be a healthy part of an individual's well-being, and fantasies will be part of an intimate partnership. With more openness and less repression, the shame around sex will decrease. Sex will then be integrated into all full, healthy relationships in any way the couple agrees to.

Ask Yourself:

What will the future of my monogamy look like?

ACKNOWLEDGEMENTS

I would like to thank Jennifer Brown, Executive Editor at Sounds True, for finding me at the Networker Symposium and encouraging me to come on board with Sounds True. She tirelessly worked through the COVID-19 pandemic to edit my chapters, while at the same time building her house, and typing with a broken wrist. She was an outspoken champion of this project from the beginning and stayed positive and supportive throughout the writing and the editing. Thank you to Laurel Szmyd, Production Editor, for her spot on edits and to Nick Small, Publicity Manager, who found me a voice at S&H six months before the book came out. And to Chloé Prusiewicz , Product Marketing Manager, and Amy Sinopoli, Contracts Manager, and Beth Conway, Foreign and Subsidiary Rights Director, for getting my audio book off the ground.

I'd like to thank some of my mentors, and only a few of them can be included here even though if I had space there would be a much larger list. Peggy Vaughan asked me to write this book years ago. When she died, she left me her notes on the future of marriage. She told me I had the voice and the vision, and wanted me to carry the torch. Thank you, Peggy. Wherever you are, I hope you like this book. To Gina Ogden, who shared her spirit, and to Janis Abrams Spring, who encourages and supports me to this day. And to my sister, Melanie Barnum, who intuitively gives me hope, and Douglas Moser, who edits me with love, and Andrew Rubenoff, who sings his heart out.

I'd also like to thank all of the brave individuals who volunteered to be interviewed for this book. Their transparency and willingness to share their stories honestly for my readers is a reflection of their integrity and how they live their lives in their relationships.

And thank you to my clients and all the couples and pods who trust me with their inner lives, who share their deepest and most private issues with me in our therapy sessions, and for teaching me that our vulnerabilities are our greatest strengths.

And to my friends who live the open monogamy life, their bravery and love knows no bounds. When I see their maturity, emotional intelligence and sexiness, I realize how important it is to be open, to stay open, and that it is absolutely possible to create the relationship of your dreams.

To my family—my children—you are the best part of my life. Thank you for making it all worth it. And finally, to Bruce, thanks for championing me through yet another book. And another lifetime.

APPENDIX:

The questionnaire below was used for each interview that is included in this book. Each interviewee was given the list of interview questions prior to our meeting and asked to share their story when we spoke by phone or in person during our interview for the *Open Monogamy*.

THE OPEN MONOGAMY INTERVIEW STRUCTURE

Thank you for being interviewed for the book *Open Monogamy*. This interview will be an essential part of my new book. I appreciate your time and how generous you are to share your story.

OPEN MONOGAMY INTERVIEW

Married:

Living Together:

Age:

Gay/Straight/Bi/Queer/Trans:

How do you want to be referred to in the book?

The book *Open Monogamy* is about the way we structure our relationships and our commitments. **I will ask you the following ten questions:**

1. How do you define your current relationship structure?

2. How did you know that traditional monogamy wasn't for you?

3. How did you approach the conversation the first time? How often do you revisit it?

4. How did this type of relationship structure develop over time?

5. Do you specifically seek out partners that will be flexible around your open monogamy?

6. Are all of your partners open? Are any of them monogamous? Are they in a consensual nonmonogamy? To whom?

7. Do other people know about your relationship agreement?

8. What is the most difficult part of your current relationship structure? What would you change?

9. What is the most meaningful part of your current relationship agreement?

10. What is the best part of your current situation?

11. Finally, is there anything else you want to add?

GLOSSARY

BDSM: A type of play that might involve bondage, discipline, sadomasochism, submission, and/or dominance.

catch-and-release agreement: An agreement between open monogamy primary partners that any outside partners will be temporary and for sex only with no lasting commitment.

closed monogamy agreement: An agreement where sexual and emotional connection stays between two specified partners.

compersion: Pleasure in their partner's happiness with someone else.

consensual nonmonogamy: *see* open monogamy

differentiated monogamy: The recognition that the two people in a couple remain individuals and do not become one person.

don't ask, don't tell policy: An agreement where a couple, explicitly or implicitly, decide not to discuss behavior that might make their partner feel jealous, hurt, or embarrassed.

equality model: A polyamorous arrangement where all partners have equal priority in the relationship.

FetLife: A website for people exploring kink and BDSM relationships.

flogging: Using a whip for sexual enjoyment.

fluid bonded agreement: An arrangement where both partners agree to have sex with someone without protection, knowing that you will share bodily fluids.

kink: Interests and behaviors outside of vanilla sex, usually including BDSM or role play activities.

kitchen table poly: An arrangement where people in primary and secondary relationships feel comfortable hanging out together.

metamour: The lover of one's partner.

Models of open monogamy: Types of open monogamous relationships including the equality model, romantic monogamy, and sexual monogamy.

monogamish: A neologism recently made popular by sex columnist Dan Savage to refer to people who adhere to social monogamy but have permeable sexual relationship boundaries (e.g., engagement in threesomes).

monogamy continuum: A spectrum of monogamy that includes the following levels: Closed, Fantasy, Emotional, Sexual, Autonomous, Independent, Unlimited, Poly, Relationship Anarchy, Detached.

nonconsensual nonmonogamy: A form of nonmonogamy without the partner's consent, or cheating.

new relationship energy (NRE): The hormones that are released when you are in the early stages of meeting a new partner and the resulting attraction and excitement that is often experienced at the beginning of a sexual and/or romantic relationship, usually lasting anywhere from three to twenty-seven months.

open monogamy: A form of partnership that permits relationships outside of the primary relationship.

outfidelity: An affair or betrayal in an open marriage.

penis-in-vagina intercourse (PIV): A traditional, hetero-focused form of sex.

pod: *see* polycule

poly: Prefix meaning "many."

polyamory: A form of open relationship involving emotional connections that may or may not include both spouses.

polycule: The group of people in a sexual, emotional, or romantic relationship network or structure.

polyfidelity relationship agreement: A multi-partner relationship agreement where if one of the partners goes outside of the group, it is a betrayal to the whole group.

primary partners: Your spouse or central, committed partner.

redline: The hard boundaries that a person is not willing change.

relationship anarchy: A nonhierarchical relationship structure that is strictly anti-monogamous, with a strong affiliation toward a lack of relational labels.

romantic monogamy: A relationship where primary partners remain emotionally true to each other but can have sexual relationships with others.

safe word: A code to indicate that a person is uncomfortable with a situation.

secondary partners: Outside partners with whom you have sex or romantic connection but are not central to your relationship.

sexual monogamy: A relationship where primary partners do not have sex with others.

solo poly: A term used to describe a person who is committed to being single but identifies with a polyamorous orientation.

squirting: The expulsion of fluid from the vulva during sex.

thruple/throuple: A polyamorous relationship between three people.

triad: *see* thruple/throuple

unicorn: A single bisexual, usually a woman, who is available for sex with a couple but is not interested in an emotional commitment.

unicorn hunter: The person in pursuit of a unicorn.

veto power: The sole power, which each partner holds and can use at any time, to decide if a relationship or behavior with any outside person should continue or if it is a threat to the primary partnership.

NOTES

Introduction

1. John Gottman, "The Science of Togetherness: Making Couples Therapy More Effective," *Psychotherapy Networker*, September/October 2017, psychotherapynetworker.org/magazine/article/1113/the-science-of-togetherness.
2. These are collective cases mingled into one for educational purposes only and to further assure their anonymity.

Chapter One

1. M.L. Haupert et al., "Prevalence of Experiences With Consensual Nonmonogamous Relationships: Findings From Two Nationally Representative Samples of Single Americans," *Journal of Sex & Marital Therapy* 43, no. 5 (June 2016): 424–40, doi.org/10.1080/00 92623X.2016.1178675.
2. Frank Newport, "In U.S., Estimate of LGBT Population Rises to 4.5%," Gallup, May 22, 2018, news.gallup.com/poll/234863/estimate-lgbt-population-rises.aspx.

Chapter Two

1. (e.g., Betzig, 1995; Goody, 1976; Lukas and Clutton-Brock, 2013; Opie, Atkinson, Dunbar, and Shultz, 2013)
2. "A History of Birth Control Methods," Katharine Dexter McCormick Library and the Education Division of Planned Parenthood Federation of America, January 2012, plannedparenthood.org/files/2613/9611/6275/History_of_BC_Methods.pdf.
3. Nena O'Neill and George O'Neill, *Open Marriage: A New Life Style for Couples* (Lanham, MD: M. Evans & Company, 1972).
4. O'Neill, *Open Marriage.*

5. Sheridan Prasso, "China's Divorce Spike Is a Warning to Rest of Locked-Down World," *Bloomberg Businessweek*, March 31, 2020, bloomberg.com/news/articles/2020-03-31/divorces-spike-in-china-after-coronavirus-quarantines.

6. Juliana Menasche Horowitz et al., "Marriage and Cohabitation in the U.S.," Pew Research Center, November 6, 2019, pewsocialtrends.org/2019/11/06/marriage-and-cohabitation-in-the-u-s.

7. Horowitz, "Marriage and Cohabitation in the U.S."

8. Elanor Barkhorn, "Cheating on Your Spouse Is Bad; Divorcing Your Spouse Is Not," *The Atlantic*, May 23, 2013, theatlantic.com/sexes/archive/2013/05/cheating-on-your-spouse-is-bad-divorcing-your-spouse-is-not/276162.

9. Peter Moore, "Young Americans Are Less Wedded to Monogamy Than Their Elders,"YouGovAmerica, October 3, 2016, today.yougov.com/topics/lifestyle/articles-reports/2016/10/03/young-americans-less-wedded-monogamy.

10. "Couples Spend an Average of $33,391 on Weddings, Incorporating Cultural, Religious and Personalized Elements, According to The Knot 2017 Real Weddings Study," The Knot Worldwide, February 14, 2018, theknotww.com/press-releases/the-knot-2017-real-weddings-study-wedding-spend.

11. *Merriam-Webster's Collegiate Dictionary*, 11th ed. (Springfield, MA: Merriam-Webster, 2003), merriam-webster.com.

12. Margalit Fox, "Nena O'Neill, 82, an Author of 'Open Marriage,' Is Dead," *New York Times*, March 26, 2006, nytimes.com/2006/03/26/books/nena-oneill-82-an-author-of-open-marriage-is-dead.html?login=smartlock&auth=login-smartlock.

13. (DePaulo and Morris, 2005; Finkel, Hui, Carswell, & Larson, 2014)

14. (Finkel et al., 2014)

15. Marta Panzeri, "Changes in Sexuality and Quality of Couple Relationship During the COVID-19 Lockdown," *Frontiers in Psychology*, September 29, 2020, doi.org/10.3389/fpsyg.2020.565823.

16. "Divorce Rate and Statistics in America," Canterbury Law Group, canterburylawgroup.com/divorce-statistics-rates.

17. Tammy Nelson, *When You're The One Who Cheats: Ten Things You Need To Know* (Lilburn, GA: RL Publishing, 2019).

18. While there has been controversy about Ashley Madison's membership, the Ernst & Young report done in 2017 indicates that every member on the site is legitimate.

19. Tammy Nelson, "The New Monogamy," TEDx Talks, youtube.com/watch?v=3JMioYaBJDc.

20. Rhonda Nicole Balzarini et al., "Comparing Relationship Quality Across Different Types of Romantic Partners in Polyamorous and Monogamous Relationships," *Archives of Sexual Behavior* 48, (May 8, 2019): 1749-1767, link.springer.com/article/10.1007/s10508-019-1416-7.

21. She-cession -needs note

22. Elinor Aspegren, "A US First? Massachusetts City Votes to Recognize Polyamorous Relationships in Domestic Partnership Policy," *USA Today*, July 3, 2020, usatoday.com/story/news/nation/2020/07/02/polyamory-massachusetts-city-somerville-relationships-us/5370718002.

23. "Cambridge Becomes 2nd US City to Legalize Polyamorous Domestic Partnerships," Polyamory Legal Advocacy Coalition, March 9, 2021, static1.squarespace.com/static/602abeb0ede5cc16ae72cc3a/t/6047c7f856dc6d6501ec8e10/1615316984759/2021-03-09+PLAC+Press+Release+revised.pdf.

24. J.M. Horowitz et al., "Marriage and Cohabitation in the U.S.," Pew Research Center, November 6, 2019, pewresearch.org/social-trends/2019/11/06/marriage-and-cohabitation-in-the-u-s.

25. Horowitz, "Marriage and Cohabitation in the U.S."

Chapter Three

1. Wednesday Martin, *Untrue: Why Nearly Everything We Believe About Women, Lust, and Infidelity Is Wrong and How the New Science Can Set Us Free* (New York: Little, Brown & Company, 2018), 166.

2. "Life Expectancy Tables," Annuity Advantage, updated June 13, 2019, annuityadvantage.com/resources/life-expectancy-tables.

3. Annelise Parkes Murphy et al., "A Prospective Investigation of the Decision to Open Up a Romantic Relationship," *Sage Journals* 12, no. 2 (April 8, 2020), journals.sagepub.com/doi/abs/10.1177/1948550619897157?journalCode=sppa&.

4. Justin K. Mogilski et al., "Jealousy, Consent, and Compersion Within Monogamous and Consensually Non-Monogamous Romantic Relationships," Archives of Sexual Behavior 48 (January 3, 2019): 1811-28, link.springer.com/article/10.1007/s10508-018-1286-4.

5. Larry J. Young, "The Neural Basis of Pair Bonding in a Monogamous Species: A Model for Understanding the Biological Basis of Human Behavior," National Academies Press (2003), ncbi.nlm.nih.gov/books/NBK97287.

6. Young, "The Neural Basis of Pair Bonding in a Monogamous Species."

7. M.L. Haupert et al., "Prevalence of Experiences With Consensual Nonmonogamous Relationships."

8. Elisabeth A. Sheff, "Solo Polyamory, Singleish, Single & Poly," Psychology Today, October 14, 2013, psychologytoday.com/us/blog/the-polyamorists-next-door/201310/solo-polyamory-singleish-single-poly.

9. Amy C. Moors et al., "Unique and Shared Relationship Benefits of Consensually Non-Monogamous and Monogamous Relationships: A Review and Insights for Moving Forward," European Psychologist 22, no. 1 (2017): 55-71, academia.edu/32015557/Unique_and_shared_relationship_benefits_of_consensually_non_monogamous_and_monogamous_relationships_A_review_and_insights_for_moving_forward.

Chapter Four

1. Margo DeMello, Feet and Footwear: A Cultural Encyclopedia (Santa Barbara, CA: ABC-CLIO, 2009).

2. Moors et al., "Unique and Shared Relationship Benefits of Consensually Non-Monogamous and Monogamous Relationships: A Review and Insights for Moving Forward."

Chapter Five

1. Nan Wise, *Why Good Sex Matters: Understanding the Neuroscience of Pleasure for a Smarter, Happier, and More Purpose-Filled Life* (Boston: Houghton Mifflin Harcourt, 2020).

2. *American Heritage Dictionary of the English Language*, 5th ed. (Boston: Houghton Mifflin Harcourt, 2011), ahdictionary.com.

Chapter Eight

1. "The Good Wife Study," Ashley Madison, 2019, ashleymadison.com/female-infidelity-statistics.

2. Anna Menta, "5 Things You Didn't Know About Female Sexuality, From Wednesday Martin's 'Untrue'," *Newsweek*, September 14, 2018, newsweek.com/wednesday-martin-untrue-women-and-sex-facts-1120752.

3. Deborah Copaken, "The 'Untrue' Woman," *The Atlantic*, September 28, 2018, theatlantic.com/entertainment/archive/2018/09/untrue-explores-female-libido/571513.

4. Arthur Aron et al., "Reward, Motivation, and Emotion Systems Associated With Early-Stage Intense Romantic Love," *Journal of Neurophysiology* 94, no. 1 (May 31, 2005): 327-37, pubmed.ncbi.nlm.nih.gov/15928068.

5. While there has been controversy about Ashley Madison's membership, the Ernst & Young report done in 2017 indicates that every member on the site is legitimate.

6. Jennifer P. Schneider et al., "Is It Really Cheating? Understanding the Emotional Reactions and Clinical Treatment of Spouses and Partners Affected by Cybersex Infidelity," *The Journal of Treatment & Prevention* 19, no. 1-2 (April 9, 2012): 123-39, tandfonline.com/doi/abs/10.1080/10720162.2012.658344.

7. Adrian J. Blow, "Infidelity in Committed Relationships II: A Substantive Review," *Journal of Marital and Family Therapy*, 31, no. 2 (April 2005): 217-33, onlinelibrary.wiley.com/doi/abs/10.1111/j.1752-0606.2005.tb01556.x.

8. Juliana Menasce Horowitz et al., "Marriage and Cohabitation in the U.S.," Pew Research Center, November 6, 2019, pewresearch.org/social-trends/2019/11/06/marriage-and-cohabitation-in-the-u-s.

9. Janis Abrahms Spring, *After the Affair: Healing the Pain and Rebuilding Trust When a Partner Has Been Unfaithful* (New York: William Morrow, 2012).

10. Tammy Nelson, *Getting the Sex You Want: Shed Your Inhibitions and Reach New Heights of Passion Together* (Beverly, MA: Quiver Books, 2012).

11. Elisabeth A. Sheff, "Failure or Transition? Redefining the 'End' of Polyamorous Relationships," December 20, 2012, elisabethsheff.com/2012/12/20/failure-or-transition-redefining-the-end-of-polyamorous-relationships.

12. Susan Wenzel, *A Happy Life in an Open Relationship: The Essential Guide to a Healthy and Fulfilling Nonmonogamous Love Life* (San Francisco: Chronicle Books, 2020).

13. Ritchie and Barker, 2006; Sheff, 2014.

14. Mogilski et al., "Jealousy, Consent, and Compersion Within Monogamous and Consensually Non-Monogamous Romantic Relationships."

15. Mogilski et al., "Jealousy, Consent, and Compersion Within Monogamous and Consensually Non-Monogamous Romantic Relationships."

16. Susan Wenzel, *A Happy Life in an Open Relationship*, 125.

Chapter Nine

1. PrEP stands for "pre-exposure prophylaxis." It is a pill that is taken every day to prevent HIV infection. The brand Truvada contains two HIV antivirals, tenofovir and emtricitabine.

Conclusion

1. Marcia C. Inhorn et al., "Egg Freezing at the End of Romance: A Technology of Hope, Despair, and Repair," *Sage Journals*, February 24, 2021, doi.org/10.1177/0162243921995892.

ABOUT THE AUTHOR

Tammy Nelson, PhD, is a TEDx speaker, a licensed counselor, a board-certified sexologist, a certified sex therapist, and a certified Imago relationship therapist. She is the author of six books, including *The New Monogamy: Redefining Your Relationship After Infidelity*. She is a frequent expert contributor in the press and has been featured in *New York Times*, *New York Times Magazine*, *Wall Street Journal*, *Rolling Stone*, *CNN*, and the *Times* and is the host of the popular podcast *The Trouble with Sex - As Dr. Tammy*, called "the NPR of sex podcasts." She is the director and founder of the Integrative Sex Therapy Institute, a training institute and think tank, and the director of the PhD program in Counseling specializing in Human Sexuality and Sex Therapy at Daybreak University in Southern California. Nelson is also a faculty member at California Institute of Integral Studies in San Francisco, a faculty presenter at the Psychotherapy Networker Symposium in Washington, DC, and returning keynote speaker at the Harvard Couples Conference in Cambridge. Learn more at drtammynelson.com.

ABOUT SOUNDS TRUE

Sounds True is a multimedia publisher whose mission is to inspire and support personal transformation and spiritual awakening. Founded in 1985 and located in Boulder, Colorado, we work with many of the leading spiritual teachers, thinkers, healers, and visionary artists of our time. We strive with every title to preserve the essential "living wisdom" of the author or artist. It is our goal to create products that not only provide information to a reader or listener but also embody the quality of a wisdom transmission.

For those seeking genuine transformation, Sounds True is your trusted partner. At SoundsTrue.com you will find a wealth of free resources to support your journey, including exclusive weekly audio interviews, free downloads, interactive learning tools, and other special savings on all our titles.

To learn more, please visit SoundsTrue.com/freegifts or call us toll-free at 800.333.9185.

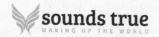